The
Hands-on Guide
to Midwifery Placements

This title is also available as an e-book.
For more details, please see www.wiley.com/buy/9781118712511
or scan this QR code:

The Hands-on Guide
to Midwifery Placements

Edited by

LUISA CESCUTTI-BUTLER
Senior Lecturer in Midwifery Bournemouth University

and

MARGARET FISHER
Associate Professor in Midwifery Plymouth University

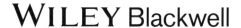
WILEY Blackwell

This edition first published 2016 © 2016 by John Wiley & Sons Ltd

Registered office:
John Wiley & Sons, Ltd, The Atrium, Southern Gate, Chichester, West Sussex, PO19 8SQ, UK

Editorial offices:
9600 Garsington Road, Oxford, OX4 2DQ, UK
The Atrium, Southern Gate, Chichester, West Sussex, PO19 8SQ, UK
350 Main Street, Malden, MA 02148-5020, USA

For details of our global editorial offices, for customer services and for information about how to apply for permission to reuse the copyright material in this book please see our website at www.wiley.com/wiley-blackwell

Library of Congress Cataloging-in-Publication Data:

The hands-on guide to midwifery placements / edited by Luisa Cescutti-Butler and Margaret Fisher.
   p. ; cm.
 Includes bibliographical references and index.
 ISBN 978-1-118-71251-1 (pbk.)
 I. Cescutti-Butler, Luisa, editor. II. Fisher, Margaret (Margaret Louise), editor.
 [DNLM: I. Midwifery–Great Britain. 2. Employment–Great Britain. 3. Preceptorship–Great Britain. WQ 160]
 RA410.7
 331.12'916182–dc23   2015029808

A catalogue record for this book is available from the British Library.

Wiley also publishes its books in a variety of electronic formats. Some content that appears in print may not be available in electronic books.

Set in 8/10 GillSansStd-Light by Thomson Digital, Noida, India
Printed and bound in Malaysia by Vivar Printing Sdn Bhd

1   2016

Contents

Contributors

Jo Coggins, RM, SOM, MSc, BSc (Hons), Dip HE (Midwifery)

Bath NHS Maternity Services, Chippenham Birthing Centre, Royal United Hospital, Bath, UK

Jo is a community midwife and Supervisor of Midwives in Wiltshire. She has a special interest in teaching and mentoring midwifery students and has published in numerous midwifery journals and texts. She lives with her husband Mark and their children Thomas and Florence.

Faye Doris, RN, RM, ADM, PGCE, MEd, SOM

School of Nursing and Midwifery, Faculty of Health and Human Sciences, Plymouth University, Devon, UK

Associate Professor (Senior Lecturer) in Midwifery, Lead Midwife for Education, Academic Lead Midwifery and Supervisor of Midwives, Faye has been a midwife teacher for many years and has led the education of midwives since joining Plymouth University in 1996. She works very closely with the maternity services in the South West and undertakes supervision of midwifery in a South West maternity unit. She is a member of the Healthcare Genetics Research Group at Plymouth. Her strength lies in the seamless way that she works across education and practice with the mother and baby being central. She enjoys working across

professional groups and promotes multi-professional working at all levels.

Henrietta Otley, RM

Family Nurse Partnership, Swindon Borough Council, Swindon, UK

After qualifying as a midwife, Hen worked at a busy teaching hospital in Bristol. After a few years, she moved into community midwifery, specialising in teenage pregnancy at a midwife-led birth centre in Wiltshire. Now she is working with the Family Nurse Partnership, a psycho-educational programme for teenagers in their first pregnancies, providing intensive home visiting services to families until the child is 2 years old. Before deciding to train as a midwife in her 30s, Hen worked in TV and radio broadcasting. She still enjoys writing, now mainly for midwifery journals.

Stella Rawnson, MA, BSc (Hons), PG Dip Ed

Midwifery & Health Professions Framework, Faculty of Health and Social Sciences, Bournemouth University, Dorset, UK

Senior Lecturer in Midwifery, Stella has spent over 20 years working as a midwife in various clinical roles. In 2002, she joined the team at Bournemouth University where she now works as senior lecturer in midwifery. She is an advocate for caseloading in practice and education, and co-leads and coordinates the student midwife caseloading initiative at Bournemouth University. Her desire to promote excellence in this respect is reflected in her research activities and area of scholarship. Her doctoral work explores women's experiences of being part of a student midwife's caseload, through hearing their personal stories.

Susan Way, PhD, MSc, PGCEA, ADM, RM

Faculty of Health and Social Sciences, Bournemouth University, Dorset, UK

Associate Professor and Lead Midwife for Education, Dr. Susan Way in her latter role leads the development, delivery and management of midwifery education programmes at Bournemouth University. She took up this role in November 2009 having previously worked for the Nursing and Midwifery Council as their Midwifery Advisor, for 8 years. Susan led a number of projects while at the NMC including the rewriting of the NMC Standards for pre-registration midwifery education as well as developing a model used to review the Local Supervising Authorities. Her PhD on women's experiences of their perineum following childbirth and has led her to continued interest in pain management following birth. Susan has presented papers at local, national and international conferences and has also published in peer-reviewed journals. In addition, she has published a book and has contributed a book chapter. In September 2013, she was elected to the RCM Board and is also Chair of the Lead Midwife for Education UK Executive Group.

Foreword

When I was first asked if I would write the foreword to a book on midwifery placements, I was somewhat bemused as to what a book with such a title might deliver or, indeed, who would be interested in what it had to say. What sprang to my mind was the complex and often exhausting allocation of students to placement areas, with dates, times and locations to facilitate the events and experiences needed to fulfil the demands of the midwifery curriculum. It felt like this could be a very dry and dull excursion into the organisation and delivery of pre-registration midwifery programmes. How wrong can one be?

The draft versions of each chapter promised exciting and important insights into the workings of undergraduate education and, more importantly, the realities and lived experiences of what it meant to be a student midwife. I was hooked and with considerable excitement, awaited the due date when the book would make its first, full-fledged appearance.

The final version has certainly delivered on its early promise and leaves me wondering why it has taken so long for a book, which is so particular and pertinent to midwifery education, to come into being? It may well be that time, culture and conditions are just right for its conception with the student central to the educational process, actively taking part in its delivery and determining not just their own future, but the future of the midwifery profession.

Midwifery placements contain nine robust and relevant chapters on important issues relating to professional practice and the role of the midwife. These range from the philosophy of midwifery care and an introduction to the rules and regulations that govern our profession to what a student needs and should consider when preparing for clinical practice. Throughout, the insight and experiences of student midwives shines through, and helpful hints provide advice and warnings for those considering or already engaged in the journey of discovery, which will hopefully lead to becoming a qualified midwife.

Having set out the rules, structures and elements of what a student midwife might encounter on their pre-registration programme, the book moves on to the challenges of learning and assessment: the acquisition of competence and those essential proficiencies that are contained and consistent with the knowledge, skills and understanding of what it is to be a midwife in the twenty-first century.

Assessment in practice, the role of the mentor and insights into both low- and high-risk placements are explored, providing important 'take home messages', which will not only excite the reader but will also make them wonder at the diversity of the educational experience. A chapter on student midwife 'caseload holding' provides an introduction to what the Australian's call 'Continuity of Care Experiences' understanding the central nature and interdependent relationships that exist between midwives and mothers, and the rich benefits it brings to those involved in such approaches to care.

What follows is a further leap in the student's journey of discovery, where wider experiences in different and diverse healthcare settings are presented, demonstrating the learning acquired through multiprofessional team work and the unique contribution different disciplines make to the health and well-being of those in our care. This moves on to 'Student Electives' with a national and global perspective, where students literally take flight, spread their wings, and reach out to discover other ways of working, other cultures and countries. The stories and experiences told by each student captivate the imagination, and made me wish that I could do it all over again.

The Hands-on Guide to Midwifery Placements, far from being a dull and boring account of an educational process, is more akin to a 'Student's Guide to the Galaxy of Professional Practice'. Throughout the book, the student contributions are both moving and beautifully written. It is both their reality and their experiences that bring to the fore the demands and difficulties, which are part and parcel of becoming a member of the midwifery profession.

Although written by very experienced clinical midwives and midwife teachers, its focus is clearly on the student midwife's road of travel. The extracts and reflections on how they felt, what they experienced and how they saw events unfolding around them make their journey come alive and will be a real help to anyone who is to embark on this adventure. This includes the qualified midwives who provide the safety net, support and sustenance necessary for the student's success and who will always be remembered.

It was a joy and a privilege to read this book and to write the foreword. I trust that it provides each and every student midwife with the help and direction they need, to fulfil their dreams of becoming a midwife, with the knowledge, skills, calm, compassion and quality of care that women seek throughout the continuum of pregnancy and childbirth.

Paul Lewis, OBE
Professor of Midwifery Practice &
Professional Development
Bournemouth University,
Dorset, UK

Preface

Student midwives spend around 50% of their under-graduate pre-registration midwifery programme in the clinical area. Going to a new placement is often a very stressful time for students as they consider: Will I 'fit in'? Do I know enough? Have I got the right skills? They may also wonder what they will learn there and how they will meet their practice assessments. The practicalities such as whether they will be able to get placement on time, how far they will have to travel and what hours they will be expected to do may also cause anxieties. Being unfamiliar with hospital environments is initially nerve wracking. If you are soon to begin your midwifery programme, we hope you will find that this handy book will offer a 'one-stop' resource, where you can access useful and practical help and information to help you adjust and get used to the surroundings as you come across different aspects of your placements. You may wish to read the book all at once as you start your very first clinical placement or dip in and out as you need throughout your programme. Each chapter contains 'top tips' obtained from current midwifery students as well as real-life student vignettes. References are provided should you wish to explore points of interest further.

Your years as a student midwife will be hard going, and at times in placement you may well think 'why am I doing this'? On other occasions you will come away full of joy after supporting a woman to birth her baby. When you are tired after a long shift in practice and you have an assignment to write the next day, hold onto these 'good times' and focus on what brought you into midwifery in the first place. This is likely to be a chance to make a difference to women in your care and a fulfilling career that enables you to be 'with woman' during her pregnancy and birth.

We hope that this book will give you helpful hints, provide a realistic perspective and encourage you as you progress along that journey. Enjoy.

Luisa Cescutti-Butler
Margaret Fisher

About the editors

Luisa Cescutti-Butler, Senior Lecturer in Midwifery, Faculty of Health and Social Sciences, Bournemouth University, RGN, RM, MA, PGDip, ENB 405/997, PhD candidate

Luisa trained as a nurse at Addington Hospital, Durban, South Africa in 1982. After several years travelling around the world, she settled in the United Kingdom and qualified as a midwife in 1990. She moved to Dorset and worked as a midwife in NHS neonatal intensive care units and in 1995 undertook the ENB 405 at Southampton University.

In 1996, Luisa moved to Salisbury NHS Foundation Trust where she undertook a variety of neonatal positions, culminating in becoming a Lecturer Practitioner in 2002, a post that was jointly shared with Bournemouth University. In 2005, Luisa was offered a full-time lecturer position at Bournemouth University. She is at present a Senior Lecturer in Midwifery and leads units under the undergraduate pre-registration midwifery programmes as well as post-registration CPD units.

Luisa completed her MA in Inter-professional Health and Social Care in 1999. Her dissertation, utilising a qualitative research approach (grounded theory), explored parents' perceptions of staff competence in a neonatal intensive care unit. Her dissertation was awarded the Eleanor Bond Prize by Salisbury NHS Foundation Trust Hospital.

Luisa's scholarship in practice focuses around examination of the newborn and all things neonatal. She facilitated a practice development project with Salisbury NHS Foundation Trust Hospital, which enabled early discharge to home of well preterm babies with community support. A current pilot project, undertaken with third-year midwifery students at Bournemouth University, is exploring the feasibility of incorporating NIPE (Newborn Infant Physical Examination) competencies into the pre-registration midwifery programme. A scoping visit to Ljubljana University, Slovenia, including conference presentation, was undertaken in 2013 to determine whether there were opportunities to expand Slovenian midwives practice to incorporate examination of the newborn.

Luisa is currently working towards her PhD at Bournemouth University. Her qualitative study using feminism as a philosophy is exploring women's experiences of caring for their late preterm infants, born between 34 and 36 + 6 completed weeks of pregnancy.

Margaret Fisher, Associate Professor in Midwifery, Programme Lead Pre-Registration Midwifery, Plymouth University RN, RM, BSc (Hons) Midwifery, PGDipHE, MSc Health Care and Educational Practice.

Margaret qualified as a nurse in South Africa and then registered as a midwife in the United Kingdom in 1988. Having worked as a clinical midwife in Exeter until 1999, she moved into education, becoming a midwifery lecturer at Plymouth University. For 3 years, she spent half her time in the Royal Devon and Exeter NHS Foundation Trust providing academic leadership for the new Placement Development Team which supported learners and mentors/practice educators from all health professions in the Trust. For the past 6 years, she has been the Programme Lead for the Pre-Registration Midwifery programme, and also spent a year as Acting Lead Midwife for Education. She has a strong belief in maintaining her own clinical practice and regularly works in the Exeter labour ward or low-risk birth centre as well as providing support to students and mentors in her role as Link Lecturer in a range of acute maternity Trusts and associated midwife-led units across the South West.

Margaret has a particular interest in practice assessment and mentorship. Her Masters dissertation explored the needs of midwifery mentors. She led a multi-professional team in a 5-year HEFCE (Higher Education Funding Council for England) funded project in the Centre for Excellence in Professional Placement Learning (CEPPL) at Plymouth University, in which a longitudinal study of students on midwifery, emergency care and social work programmes was conducted to explore assessment of practice. She is currently part of a small team of senior midwifery academics who have been undertaking a scoping activity of grading of practice through the UK Lead Midwives for Education UK Executive group. These findings were presented at the International Confederation of Midwives 30th Triennial Congress in Prague in June 2014, and have recently been submitted for publication. She has presented at a number of national and international conferences on the topic of practice assessment and mentorship, and several of her publications are referred to in this book.

Acknowledgements

This book is dedicated to all the midwifery students from Bournemouth University and Plymouth University who so generously provided us with top tips for placement and willingly shared their vignettes. Two students need a particular mention: Clare Shirley who created two original cartoons depicting aspects of being a midwife and Hugo Beaumont who designed the 'which hat am I wearing today' image. Thanks are due to Professor Paul Lewis OBE for his foreword and the chapter authors: Dr. Sue Way, Hen Otley, Jo Coggins, Stella Rawnson and Faye Doris for their fabulous contributions. I (LC-B) would like to thank Madeline Hurd (formerly Associate Commissioning Editor on the health sciences education books team at Wiley-Blackwell) for taking the idea of the book forward and for getting my co-editor Margaret Fisher on board. It has been a pleasure working with Margaret. We would also like to thank James Schultz (Project Editor) and James Watson (Associate Commissioning Editor) at Wiley-Blackwell for their help and support in bringing this book out. In addition Margaret and I acknowledge the support we've had from our respective universities (Plymouth & Bournemouth) who gave us time to collaborate on this book. We hope both current and future students will enjoy it. Lastly we also have to acknowledge and thank the women and their partners, midwives and the midwifery students who participated in the many photographs, vignettes and 'top tips' within this book: Rebecca Allum, Emma Barton, Hugo Beaumont, Laura Brier, Jasmine Buckmaster, Gayle Callaby, Rachael Callan, Aimee Cannings, Kerry Coleman, Caroline Cook, Sophie Denning, Lou Ellis, Alex Evans, Eloise Fanning, Becky Fry, Amanda Gill, Diane Humphries, Jo Lake, Jenny McAdam, Kerrie-Anne Mcindoe, Georgia Moffatt, Keri Morter, Laura Marks, Arlene Oram, Jenna Penhale, Tobi Penhale, Sian Ridden, Luzie Schroter, Zoe Shama, Victoria Shaw, Clare Shirley, Caitlin Taylor, Molly Taylor, Dave Waldrin, Kirsty Waldrin, Millie Westwood, and Laura Woodhouse.

Luisa Cescutti-Butler
Margaret Fisher

List of abbreviations

AA	Academic Advisor (a term which may be used for the midwifery academic who supports you academically, clinically and for personal/pastoral issues)
AEI	Approved Education Institution (or University)
AIMS	Association for Improvements in the Maternity Services
BNF	British National Formulary (the 'bible' of medicines in the United Kingdom)
BP	blood pressure
BSc	Bachelor of Science
BU	Bournemouth University
CC	credit card
CDS	Central Delivery Suite (may also be known as labour ward)
CEPPL	Centre for Excellence in Professional Placement Learning (Government-funded Centre for Excellence in Teaching and Learning at Plymouth University)
CMACE	Centre for Maternal and Child Enquiries (investigates mortality; now replaced by MBRRACE)
CPD	continuous professional development
CQC	Care Quality Commission (monitors standards of NHS service providers)
C/S	Caesarean section
CTG	cardiotocography (electronic monitoring of fetal heart rate and uterine contractions)
CV	curriculum vitae
DBS	Disclosure and Barring Service (criminal background screening required for professions in which contact with the public is required; in the case of midwifery and similar professions, this entails an enhanced screening which will flag up any previous criminal cautions or convictions)
DOB	date of birth

DoH/DH	Department of Health
EBM	expressed breast milk
EDD	estimated due date
ESC	Essential Skills Clusters (key skills needed by midwives, identified by the NMC)
EU	European Union
FCO	Foreign and Commonwealth Office
FH	fetal heart
FTP	Fitness to Practise (a process used for registrants by the NMC and required to be included in pre-registration midwifery and nursing programmes)
GP	general practitioner
Hb	haemoglobin
HELLP	a syndrome comprising '**H**aemolysis (breaking down of red blood cells), **E**levated **L**iver enzymes, **L**ow **P**latelet count (a clotting factor)' – a very serious condition which can occur in a pregnant woman who has pre-eclampsia
HIV	human immunodeficiency virus
HMSO	Her Majesty's Stationery Office (Government publishing department)
HOM	Head of Midwifery (midwife responsible for the maternity services in a trust)
HOOP (trial)	'hands on or poised' (a trial conducted in the late 1990s which compared outcomes if the midwife had her/his hands actively positioned on the fetal head and perineum during birth or did not undertake any physical intervention)
HR	Human Resource department
ICM	International Confederation of Midwives
ICSI	intra-cytoplasmic sperm injection (injection of a single sperm into an ovum)
IM	independent midwifery (self-employed midwives)
IMUK	Independent Midwives United Kingdom (organisation of independent midwives)
ItP	Intention to Practise (annual notification currently required by midwives to licence them to practise)

IV/i.v.	intravenous (route for medication or fluids)
IVF	in vitro fertilisation (fertilisation of the ovum takes place in a laboratory setting and the embryo is then transferred to the mother's uterus)
LOA	left occipitoanterior (the three abbreviations (LOA, LOP and LOT) are terms used in relation to the position of the unborn baby: the *presentation* is usually cephalic (known as baby has its head down); the *denominator* indicates the position, that is when the baby is head down, the *denominator* is the occiput (back of the baby's head); if the baby is in a breech position, the sacrum (bottom) is the *denominator* and if the baby's face is presenting, the chin is known as the *denominator*. The *position* of the unborn baby refers to the relationship of the denominator to areas of a woman's pelvis which are left and right anterior, left and right lateral and left and right posterior. Therefore, when a baby is presenting head down (cephalic), the occiput is the fixed point (denominator) and the position of the unborn baby is described as LOA, LOP etc.)
LOP	left occipitoposterior
LOT	left occiput transverse (not commonly used nowadays but may still be used in practice by some midwives)
LSA	Local Supervising Authority (is responsible for ensuring that statutory supervision of all midwives, as required in the Nursing and Midwifery Order (2001) and the Nursing and Midwifery Council's (NMC) Midwives rules and standards (2012) is exercised to a satisfactory standard within its geographical boundary)
LW	Labour Ward (may also be known as Central Delivery Suite or CDS)
MBRRACE	Mothers and Babies: Reducing Risk through Audits and Confidential Enquiries (has taken over from CMACE)
MCAs	maternity care assistants (work with women and midwives. Undertake tasks and care on the maternity wards and in the community. Always work under the direction of a midwife. May have taken on extra study such as NVQs: national vocational qualifications)
MINT	Midwives in Teaching Project (study commissioned by the NMC to look at preparation of students to become midwives and the role of the midwife teacher)
MSLC	Maternity Services Liaison Committee
MSWs	maternity support workers (similar role to MCAs)
NCT	National Childbirth Trust
NHS	National Health Service

NICE	National Institute for Health and Care Excellence
NMC	Nursing and Midwifery Council (the professional regulatory body for nurses, midwives and health visitors in the United Kingdom)
NQM	newly qualified midwife
OAR	Ongoing Achievement Record (used to log a student's clinical and academic progress)
OSCE	Objective Structured Clinical Examination – a practical assessment commonly used in health care programmes in which a simulated situation is provided for the student to demonstrate their clinical skills and underpinning knowledge. Stations may be 'active' (e.g. the student is required to demonstrate clinical skills or answer a viva etc.) or 'passive' (e.g. the student may be given a set of notes/blood results/cardiotocograph to interpret and document findings)
PAD	portfolio of academic development (used in some universities to log a student's clinical and academic progress)
PHSO	Parliamentary Health Ombudsman
PIN	Personal Identifying Number (the number the NMC gives you when you first register with them on qualification as a midwife or nurse)
PND	postnatal depression
POPPI	Plymouth Online Practice Placement Information (website readily accessible providing useful information for students and mentors relating to practice placements, guidelines and policies and mentorship skills)
PPH	postpartum haemorrhage (vaginal bleeding after the birth of the baby)
PREP	Post Registration Education and Practice (ongoing professional development required of registered nurses and midwives, soon to be replaced by revalidation)
PROMPT	PRactical Obstetric Multi-Professional Training – Winter et al. 2012 (a manual widely used by student midwives and other professionals to support practice in obstetric emergencies)
PT	personal tutor (a term which may be used for the midwifery academic who supports you academically, clinically and for personal/pastoral issues)
PU	Plymouth University
RCM	Royal College of Midwives
RCN	Royal College of Nurses

ROA	right occipitoanterior (see explanation provided around LOA)
ROP	right occipitoposterior (as above)
ROT	right occiput transverse (not commonly used nowadays but may still be used in practice by some midwives)
SCPHN	Specialist Community and Public Health Nurse
SOM/SoM	Supervisor of Midwives (currently a statutory role with the aim of protecting the public)
SRM/SROM	spontaneous rupture of membranes. The membranes hold together a fluid-filled bag (also known as the amniotic sac) which surrounds and protects the unborn baby. SRM is also called 'breaking of the waters'. Membranes can break by themselves (as at the beginning of labour or during labour itself) or a midwife may break them (ARM or artificial rupture of membranes) during labour to 'speed things up', although this is debated in the literature. The best time for the membranes to break would be just before the baby is born.
SpLD	specific learning difference (e.g. dyslexia, dyspraxia and dyscalculia)
SU	Student Union (a university-based group which acts on behalf of its students; may or not be part of the National Union of Students)
SWOT	strengths, weaknesses, opportunities and threats (a well-recognised framework for self-appraisal)
TENS	transcutaneous electrical nerve stimulator – a self-administered method of analgesia used to promote endorphin production
USS	ultrasound scan (scan usually undertaken at around 12 weeks of pregnancy, known as the dating scan, and will provide a EDD and again at 18–20 weeks which checks the unborn baby for any abnormalities. Sometimes later in pregnancy, women will be sent for further scans to check for growth of the unborn baby)
UK	United Kingdom
VBAC	'vaginal birth after caesarean' (a woman who has previously had a caesarean section has a trial of labour with the intention of a normal birth)
vs	versus

Chapter 1
INTRODUCTION TO MIDWIFERY AND THE PROFESSION

Susan Way

Introduction

Starting your midwifery programme is an exciting time and a key element of your role is being 'with woman'. One of the aims of this chapter is to explore various beliefs about how care should be provided, with the aim of starting you off thinking about the kind of midwife you would like to be. It explores philosophies and models of care, including the 6C's and how, through the use of appropriate language, you always keep women at the centre of your care. The latter half of this chapter helps you understand the role of the Nursing and Midwifery Council (NMC), the regulatory body that is responsible for setting the rules and regulations that govern our practice as midwives, and how these will impact on you the moment you become a student midwife. They will shape the knowledge and skills you acquire, but more importantly the way you behave and what is expected of you by the public.

Philosophy of care

What is the practice of midwifery?

Midwifery care is practised by many different people across the globe such as qualified midwives, obstetricians, support workers, family doctors and traditional birth attendants. The quality of care will be different depending on the training or lack of training that the person has received. Who and how they were taught, their skills will accordingly shape the way they think and practise midwifery.

Introduction to philosophy

Philosophy is a way of thinking which has a common understanding and is shared by a group of people or from personal experience – forming an individual perspective. Philosophy is, therefore, a particular way of thinking. A philosophy of care in a midwifery context is how

The Hands-on Guide to Midwifery Placements, First Edition.
Edited by Luisa Cescutti-Butler and Margaret Fisher.
© 2016 John Wiley & Sons, Ltd. Published 2016 by John Wiley & Sons, Ltd.

healthcare professionals such as midwives believe care should be provided to women, their babies and families.

A significant report in 1993 commonly referred to as 'Changing Childbirth' or Cumberlege report, named after the Chair of the Committee, Baroness Cumberlege (DoH 1993) detailed for the first time that care provided to pregnant women should be kinder, more welcoming and more supportive. Women and their families should be at the centre of maternity services, which should be planned and provided with their interests and those of their babies in mind. Other reports have continued to drive this policy forward (DoH 2007, 2009, 2010; The Maternity Services Action Group 2011). 'Changing Childbirth' (1993) offered a different way of thinking about how care should be provided, and supported a particular philosophy that many midwives were trying to practise or aspire to.

Before the 'Changing Childbirth' report was published, evidence was beginning to show that women were becoming increasingly dissatisfied with maternity services and that women wanted more continuity and individualised care (Garcia 1982). As more women birthed in hospitals (up to 98% by the end of the 1970s), care had become fragmented and women were subjected to many, often unnecessary, interventions, without any thought of individual circumstances, needs or experiences. For example, all women would have been given an enema at the beginning of labour, because it was believed that this reduced the amount of soiling, the length of labour and the risk of infection. Romney and Gordon's (1981) important piece of research challenged whether enemas were actually needed and so eventually it was stopped, but it took some time. In the same period, care offered to women began to be task focussed with different midwives being involved with specific activities or aspects of care. This meant that women would be seen by a range of midwives during the antenatal, labour and postnatal periods; the end result was that women were unable to build a trusting relationship with 'their' midwife. Thompson (1980 cited in Bryar 1991 p49) describes this conflict with the following statement:

> 'we [midwives] have become assembly-line workers with each midwife doing a little bit to each woman who passes by'.

Two opposing philosophies

The 'Changing Childbirth' report and subsequent policy initiatives emphasise the need to put women at the heart of maternity care taking into account their individual social, spiritual and psychological needs and wishes. The other viewpoint puts task-orientated care and the needs of the organisation above those of the woman; progressing large numbers of women through a factory-like system to achieve efficiency and productivity.

The social or physiological model

Acknowledging the woman as a whole person is often talked about as holistic care, and the philosophy related to this is sometimes referred to as a social or physiological model or approach. Supporters of this philosophy would argue that childbirth is a normal physiological event, where the progress of pregnancy, birth and the postnatal period is seen as normal and not defined as being at the risk of something going wrong (Royal College of Midwives 1997). Routine practices and interventions such as withholding food and drink from women in labour are not used as they are seen as unnecessary in improving the health of women and their babies. Women and midwives are viewed as partners in care, sharing knowledge to enable women to make their own choices based on accurate and unbiased information. A trusting relationship is built between midwives and women, empowering women to be in control of their own birth experience. Women are the focus of care, with midwives listening and responding to their needs. The approach aims to increase women's independence or autonomy over the whole childbirth experience (DoH 2004, 2012). An example of a student midwife's philosophy is shared below. Mille wrote this philosophy for her caseloading module and it reflects the care she provides to women – not only those within her caseload but all women with whom Millie comes into contact.

Vignette 1.1 Philosophy of care

My philosophy of midwifery practice stems from my personal values. These are to treat all individuals, irrespective of background, with kindness, dignity and respect. To me, midwifery is about guiding each woman through a normal, but changing, stage in her life. In order to form a meaningful relationship, I think it is important to have a compassionate and empathetic approach from the first point of contact which would entail understanding any particular additional needs the woman may have. The power of a smile is underestimated; it can help relieve anxieties from the outset, showing that you are friendly and want to be there with the woman.

I believe that my care of a woman must be founded on a mutually trusting relationship wherein she feels both safe with, and confident in me at all times. I believe that a trusting bond between the woman and the midwife is most likely to develop from the midwife's competent and committed care, which is non-judgemental, and tailored to her needs regardless of culture, age, disability, or sexual orientation.

I believe the woman will be empowered to make informed choices and to feel comfortable in doing so if the midwife is honest, open minded and quietly assistive. This gives the woman control over, and confidence in her body and its ability to take her through her journey of pregnancy and childbirth. In this way, midwifery becomes a woman-centred approach, which is fundamental to good practice.

(continued)

Holistic care is very important to me. In addition to the woman's physical needs, any psychological, social and emotional needs should always be addressed to enable high-quality health care. This care might be expanded to meet public health needs, such as education about adapting to motherhood, and about weight management.

Millie Westwood
Third-year student, Bournemouth University, Dorset, UK
Reproduced with permission of Millie Westwood

Medical model

At the other end of the scale is the focus on preventing or reducing the risk of something going wrong. This requires an approach where statistics and medical intervention are considered more important and is often referred to as a medical model of care, with an understanding that pregnancy and birth is potentially risky and that childbirth can only be classed as a normal once the outcome is known (Walsh et al. 2004; van Teijlingen 2005). The body is divided up and viewed as separate systems such as the circulatory system, the reproductive system or the nervous system, resulting in care being delivered according to the system under inspection rather than the body as a whole. An example would be the differing views towards pain in labour. A physiological approach may mean that it is important for a woman to experience this, viewing it as a way of connecting with her soon to be born baby and that labour contractions are a life-giving force to enable the birth to take place. The medical model would however see this as a problem which needs to be cured; pain relief such as an epidural would therefore be offered routinely.

Although referred to as the medical model, it is not always or only practised by doctors but many midwives also support this view. Medical or technological interventions become important in managing any potential risk that may be harmful to the progress of pregnancy or labour and birth. The term 'risk' has more recently appeared in the midwifery literature, with concepts such as 'antenatal screening for risk of abnormality' and 'risk criteria for midwife led care' being used (Thomas 2003). Interventions in labour to manage such risks include birthing in hospital, induction of labour, rupturing membranes, episiotomy and caesarean section; these are undertaken in the belief that the health of the woman and her baby will be improved.

Comparing the models

Further differences between the two models are seen when comparing how success is defined in terms of birth outcome. With the physiological model, factors are taken into account such as given in Fig. 1.1.

Even if the woman required an operative procedure to birth her baby the above needs should still be met. The success indicators are fairly broad and

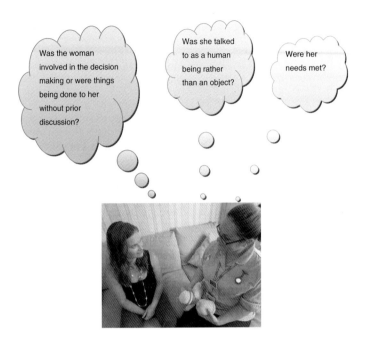

Figure 1.1 Physiological model: factors to consider.

relate very much to the experience of the woman and her family. The indicators of success for the physiological model demonstrate that social, cultural and psychological factors all have an influence on outcome that can impact on the birth experience well beyond the completion of birth. Successful outcomes of birth within the medical model are talked about in relation to illness or injury (often referred to as morbidity) as well as mortality – the death of a woman or newborn baby. Numbers or statistics are often used to demonstrate results of causes and cures for specific disorders.

The following quotes taken from a report published by the Care Quality Commission (CQC) highlight two women's contrasting experiences:

'we found out a few days before my baby was due that he was breech [bottom first rather than head]. Various options were made available to us but we chose a planned Caesarean Section. All of the staff I came into contact with were very kind and explained everything'

CQC (2013:14)

"Due to me not being listened to and being ignored when I was telling the midwives

I felt labour had started. I was left in a room with other women and not checked for $4^{1/2}$ hours even though I went to them 3 times to tell them I felt my baby was coming. After me struggling to their desk in the early hours and arguing, they eventually checked me and discovered the head was there. I had given them many opportunities to check earlier and asked for a private room but this was ignored leaving me alone with 2 other women sharing my room = DISGUSTING!'

CQC (2013:24)

The two opposing models of midwifery care expressed above are extreme ends of a spectrum and some midwives' practise would incorporate elements from both. Categorising the approaches to care in terms of models provides a way of understanding people's thinking and can be considered a way of simplifying aspects of a complex world (Ireland & van Teijlingen 2013). Our philosophical style to the practice of midwifery may well have been influenced by our view on life. This can impact on the way we see the world and so start to use the model in our own lives and subsequently in our practise as midwives.

Women's views of maternity care

Negative feedback reinforces the view from the Department of Health that women should be at the heart of maternity care (2004, 2005) and that midwives have an integral role in developing woman-centred care (DoH 2010). The Chief Nurse for England, Jane Cummings refers to the 6Cs of care, compassion, competence, communication, courage and commitment and how these can improve the culture of care we give (NHS Commissioning Board 2012). Using these 6Cs, midwives can make a significant contribution to high quality, compassionate and excellent health and well-being outcomes for women across all settings.

Recently Renfrew et al. (2014: 2), in order to assess the quality of midwifery care from a global perspective, defined the practice of midwifery as:

'skilled, knowledgeable and compassionate care for childbearing women, newborn infants and families across the continuum throughout pre-pregnancy, pregnancy, birth, postpartum and the early weeks of life. Core characteristics include optimising normal biological, physiological, social and cultural processes of reproduction and early life; timely prevention and management of complications; consultation with and referral to other services; respect for women's individual circumstances and views; and working in partnership with women to strengthen women's own capabilities to care for themselves and their families'.

Many of the core characteristics reflect the 6Cs as well as a philosophy that respects the individual contribution that women make to their own care.

A humanising values framework has been developed to show how these principles can be incorporated into the midwifery care you will be providing

Table 1.1 Dimensions of humanisation.

Forms of humanisation	Forms of dehumanisation
Insiderness: experiencing the world through mood, feeling and emotion	Objectification: seeing women with a list of problems rather than a holistic person
Agency: having freedom to make choices	Passivity: not enabled to make true, informed choice
Uniqueness: being individual and having unique characteristics	Homogenisation: fitting people into boxes such as, the obese woman, the smoker
Togetherness: belonging within a community of care giver, family and friends	Isolation: isolated through negative relationships with the midwife(s), family and friends
Sense making: value the experience of women and support them to make sense of it	Loss of meaning: ignoring experiences because they are different, difficult to accept or do not have the time to listen
Personal journey: acknowledge the childbirth journey as part of a bigger life event	Loss of personal journey: not recognising the impact of childbirth as a life event
Sense of place: environments offer familiarity, comfort and safety	Dislocation: environments lack privacy and dignity that can sometimes be frightening and inflexible
Embodiment: recognising the woman within their psychological, social and socio-cultural context	Reductionism: stereotyping women into particular behaviours such as those who construct a birth plan being seen as 'difficult'

Adapted from the dimensions of humanisation (Todres et al. 2009).

(Todres et al. 2009). There are eight themes and the diagram given in Table 1.1 demonstrates dimensions of humanisation/dehumanisation. During your time in practice reflect on the dimensions of humanisation to help develop the care you offer into being woman-centred, compassionate and caring.

Top ten tips for what women want from their midwives/ student midwives

Luisa Cescutti-Butler

AIMS (Association for Improvements in the Maternity Services) a volunteer organisation was founded in 1960 by

Sally Willington. Her story, describing her antenatal and birth experience was published in a national newspaper, which resulted in many other women also complaining about their experiences. Thus, AIMS was 'born' and as a campaigning pressure group, its underlying premise is based on believing that change for women in childbirth comes from supporting midwives as autonomous practitioners in their own right, and who should be the lead carer for women and babies throughout the childbirth continuum (AIMS 2012; DoH 2010). Over the last 54 years, AIMS have campaigned for changes in maternity services, and as a result of these campaigns have collected a rich database of women's experiences which have all shown similar themes. These themes have enabled AIMS, and now us, to better understand what women would like from midwives as they journey through pregnancy, birth and beyond (AIMS 2012). The themes represented in Fig. 1.2 as top ten tips are primarily aimed at midwives; however, they will be equally relevant to you as a student midwife.

Watch your language

Luisa Cescutti-Butler

Communication is at the heart of everything we do as humans. As midwives we spend much of our working day sharing and communicating with pregnant women and their families, or with our colleagues. Throughout all interactions we need to consider our use of language. Inappropriate words and phrases used by healthcare professionals may undermine a woman's confidence in herself, and more specifically in her ability to birth her baby and be a mother (Robertson 1999; Simkin et al. 2012). This section will highlight some of the common phrases you may hear midwives and others use whilst in placement, and provide you with alternative suggestions. By being mindful of the language you use when interacting with women you are well on your way to being 'with woman'.

1 Midwives are commonly heard referring to women in their care as 'my ladies' or 'my women' (Simkin et al. 2012). Mary Stewart, in a paper where a number of authors discuss concepts around 'language of birth', dislikes the use of the words 'lady' or 'ladies' to describe women. These two particular phrases represent in her opinion, the concept of a woman belonging to her husband, a possession and defined by her relationship to her husband. She also objects to the use of 'my' which implies a relationship where the balance of power lies with the healthcare professional and not with the woman (Simkin et al. 2012). Other expressions you may hear being used frequently by midwives are: "I delivered Mrs Blogs baby", "I had a C/S last night", "I had twins last week", "I had a PPH today" (Robertson 1999; Hunter 2006). These phrases suggest ownership of the birthing process, the woman is just the 'problem' and goes against the midwifery philosophy of woman-centred care (Lichtman 2013).

2 Imagine you are in the early stages of labour and experiencing a lot of discomfort during your labour contractions and are told by a midwife "You are only in early labour" or "you are still only

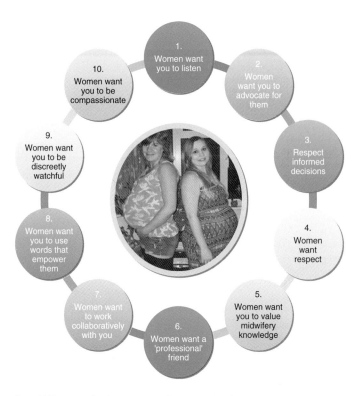

Figure 1.2 Top ten tips for what women want from their midwives/student midwives.

5 cm''. How would you feel? Perhaps you were once 'that woman'! Women are very receptive during their labour; choose your words carefully to describe their progress. 'Still' and 'only' may make them feel negative about what they have achieved so far and for what is to come (Robertson 1999).

3 'The section in bed '4', the induction in room '1', 'she's 3 cm', 'she's contracting', are terms which demote women to a 'series of body parts' (Simkin et al. 2012). This, in effect, is a reductionist approach to viewing and referring to women and reflects a biomedical model of care. It is not reflective of a holistic approach, it is patronizing and the language reflects an environment that is medicalised and technical and women are there to have 'things done to them' (Carboon 1999).

4 Consider the impression these phrases convey 'failure to progress', 'incompetent cervix', 'trial of scar', 'inadequate contractions'. Do they inspire confidence in a woman's ability to birth? Terms such as these indicate women need to be closely observed and regularly monitored during labour and may even require 'fixing' at some point (Simkin et al. 2012; Hunter 2006; Pollard 2011).

5 What does the word 'patient' mean to you? If you are a student on the shortened midwifery programme and are a registered nurse, you will need to adjust your conceptual thinking around this term. 'Patient' is a term which suggests illness; it also suggests obedience and an acceptance that care is done to you (Hunter 2006). Let us not forget that some women do become patients because they develop complications either during their pregnancy or post birth, so it may be entirely appropriate to refer to them as patients. However for healthy women the environment of birth should not determine their status. Women who birth at home are seldom referred to as 'patients', the same respect should be accorded to women who have babies in hospital. Interestingly, the first ever national Dignity Survey of Women's Experiences of Childbirth in the United Kingdom highlighted that women who gave birth in hospitals experienced less choice and respectful care than those who gave birth in birth centres or at home (Prochaska 2013).

So is there a language of birth? We know what women want! They would like midwives and the wider team to use positive language (AIMS 2012). Choosing our words carefully and spoken at the right time can positively enhance a woman's experience of pregnancy and childbirth. Consider replacing 'delivery' with 'birth' (Robertson 1999). Reflect on the expression 'the section in bed 4'. How would that make you feel if you were that woman? The words are degrading and impersonal – instead why not say 'the woman in bed 4 has had a baby' and also remember that she has undergone major abdominal surgery and all the issues that go alongside an operative birth (Simkin et al. 2012) (Fig. 1.3).

It is not always easy to change the words we have used over many years and this is nicely portrayed by a midwife responding to a blog on the importance of language written by Sheena Byrom. The midwife describes how she initially felt awkward saying 'attending a birth' instead of 'delivering a baby', but soon got used to it (Byrom 2013). Women birth their own babies; midwives guide and facilitate the process (Lichtman 2013). As Hunter (2006) elegantly reminds us, women give birth and pizzas are delivered!

As an educationalist, I encourage students at all levels to embrace language that is women-centred. I avoid words that are not women-friendly in my teaching resources and when discussing or debating midwifery issues with students. I try not to refer to students that I tutor as 'my students' and am also careful to avoid referring to particular students as 'the student'. This strategy I hope serves as an example of how students themselves should be mindful of the use of their own language both with women and when discussing women with

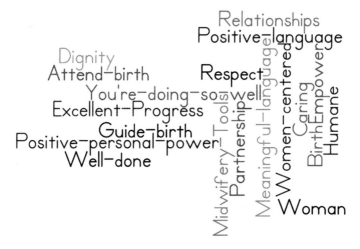

Figure 1.3 Positive language wordle.

colleagues in placement. We need to be constantly aware of the language we use and take responsibility for our words so that we can transform and enhance care for women (Simkin et al. 2012).

What is a midwife?

Sue Way

The International Confederation of Midwives (ICM 2011) offers the definition given in Fig. 1.4.

In the United Kingdom, the title 'midwife' is protected by law, which means it can only be used by a person who is registered on the midwives' part of the NMC register.

The nursing and midwifery council (NMC)

Having researched your chosen career in midwifery, you will have quickly realised that between 50% and 60% of your programme will take place in clinical practice. The variety of clinical experience alongside the academic content of the programme is set by the NMC, the regulatory body for nurses and midwives in the United Kingdom (England, Northern Ireland, Scotland and Wales). The NMC is an organisation set up by Parliament, whose main aim is to safeguard the health and well-being of the public by ensuring a high standard of care to those

> "A midwife is a person who has successfully completed a midwifery education programme that is duly recognized in the country where it is located and that is based on the ICM Essential Competencies for Basic Midwifery Practice and the framework of the ICM Global Standards for Midwifery Education; who has acquired the requisite qualifications to be registered and/or legally licensed to practice midwifery and use the title 'midwife'; and who demonstrates competency in the practice of midwifery"

Figure 1.4 ICM definition of a midwife.

who need and use the services of midwives and nurses. The organisation:

■ safeguards the health and well-being of the public;

■ sets standards of education, training, conduct and performance so that nurses and midwives can deliver high-quality healthcare consistently throughout their careers;

■ ensures that nurses and midwives keep their skills and knowledge up to date and uphold the NMC professional standards and

■ has clear and transparent processes to investigate nurses and midwives who fall short of the NMC's standards.

The NMC publishes rules, standards and guidance for nurses, midwives, employers, students and members of the public to understand how the above is achieved; however, the following are of particular interest

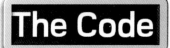

The Code is the foundation of high-quality midwifery practice and midwives must safeguard the health and well-being of women, babies and their families. If a midwife's conduct, performance or ethics fall below the standard set by the Code, this may call into question their fitness to practice and jeopardise their registration.

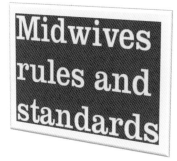

Midwifery practice is governed by these rules and all midwives must adhere to them.

Figure 1.5 NMC publications of interest to student midwives. (Source: NMC: www.nmc-uk.org.)

to midwives and you as a student in training (Fig. 1.5). Should you wish to read them in full please look at the reference list for the complete details of each publication.

A further document which may be of interest to you is Standards for pre-registration midwifery education (NMC 2009) which outlines the standards of education and training necessary for you to qualify as a midwife (Table 1.2). As this book goes to print, the NMC is undertaking a review of the pre-registration education standards, so they may look different in the near future. It is always

useful to look at the NMC website on a regular basis to find out what is happening and what is new.

The NMC holds a register of all nurses and midwives who are entitled to practise, which can be viewed by any member of the public. Registration with the NMC provides the nurse or midwife with a license to practise (more can be read about this in Chapter 9). Once you have successfully completed your midwifery programme, signed your declaration of good health and good character form and the Lead Midwife for Education has recommended to the NMC that you

Table 1.2 Standards for pre registration midwifery education (Adapted from NMC 2009).

Standards	Scope of standards
Standards for the lead midwife for education	
Standard 1	Appointment of the lead midwife for education
Standard 2	Development, delivery and management of midwifery education programmes
Standard 3	Signing the supporting declaration of good health and good character
Standards for admission to, continued participation in, pre-registration midwifery programmes	
Standard 4	General requirements related to selection for and continued participation in approved programmes, and entry to the register
Standard 5	Interruptions to pre-registration midwifery education programmes
Standard 6	Admission with advanced standing
Standard 7	Transfer between approved education institutions
Standard 8	Stepping off and stepping on to pre-registration midwifery education programmes
Standards for the structure and nature of pre-registration midwifery programmes	
Standard 9	Academic standard of programme
Standard 10	Length of programme
Standard 11	Student support
Standard 12	Balance between clinical practice and theory
Standard 13	Scope of practice
Standard 14	Supernumerary status during clinical practice
Standard 15	Assessment strategy
Standard 16	On-going record of achievement
Standard 17	Competencies required to achieve the NMC standards
The Essential Skills Clusters	

are eligible for registration, you will be able to apply to join the midwives' part of the NMC register. Currently, in order to be fit to practise as a midwife you must also have notified your Intention to Practice (ItP) to the Local Supervising Authority, paid your annual registration fee and have an appropriate professional indemnity arrangement. Professional indemnity insurance means that if you in some way cause harm to a woman or her baby because of negligence then the woman will be able to recover any compensation she is entitled to (www.nhsemployers.org). If you work within the NHS, the NHS will have an appropriate indemnity arrangement in place for you. If you are self-employed you need to have your own arrangements in place. As a self-employed midwife, sourcing professional indemnity insurance may not be easy as highlighted by Lewis (2014). In January 2015, the NMC made the decision to remove statutory supervision from its legal framework. Once the legislation is amended there will be a number of changes, one of which is likely to be that midwives will no longer have to submit an annual ItP as referred to above'.

Having registered with the NMC, you are able to practise as a midwife, but learning does not stop there. Every 3 years the NMC requires you to complete a Notification of Practice (NoP) declaration stating that you have met the Post-registration Education and Practice Requirements (PREP). Revalidation will replace the PREP requirement in 2016. Revalidation means that you will be required to declare that you have

■ met the requirement for practice hours and continuing professional development (CPD);

■ reflected on your practice, based on the minimum requirements of the Code, using feedback from women, relatives, colleagues and others and

■ received confirmation from a third party that your evidence is acceptable, such as your manager.

The NMC and midwifery education

The NMC does not provide the education and training for student midwives; this is the responsibility of an approved education institution (AEI), more commonly known as a University. The University works in partnership with service partners (usually NHS Trusts) who provide clinical placements. The NMC calls this joint collaboration of the University and service partners 'programme providers'. The programme providers interpret the standards and develop a curriculum (programme of study) that meets national and local need. Often members of the public such as women who have recently given birth, or members of lay organisations such as the local Maternity Services Liaison Committee (MSLC) or breastfeeding support groups are also involved in the development of the curriculum.

The standards set by the NMC for pre-registration midwifery education have to meet the requirements of the European Union Directive 2013/35/EU of the European Parliament and of the Council (2013) on the recognition of professional qualifications. This ensures that all members of the EU provide a training programme of a similar standard. An example of some key practice skills can be found in Table 1.3. This enables midwives across Europe to freely move from one-member states to another without further training.

Although the standards set by the NMC are national standards – they are required to be met by all universities

Table 1.3 The European Directive 2013/35/EU: key practise skills.

Advising of pregnant women, involving at least 100 prenatal examinations

Supervision and care of at least 40 women in labour

Initiation into care in the field of medicine & surgery, initiation includes theory & clinical practice

Students should personally carry out at least 40 deliveries, if 40 cannot be achieved it may be reduced to 30 provided the student participates actively in 20 further deliveries

Active participation with breech deliveries. If not possible practice may be simulated

Care of women with pathological conditions in the field of gynaecology and obstetrics

Performance of episiotomy and initiation into suturing through theory & clinical practice

Observation and care of the newborn, requiring special care, including preterm, postterm and ill newborn babies

Supervision, care and examination of at least 100 women and healthy newborn infants

Supervision and care of 40 women at risk in pregnancy, labour or postnatal period

across the United Kingdom offering a pre-registration programme – there will be individual variation to meet the needs of the local population. For example, the practice environment that students link to from a particular University may have a large number of women who are immigrants with specific cultural and health needs which may not be as evident in another University's area. This does not mean the latter University excludes the teaching of cultural diversity, but its application to practice may be different.

Before a pre-registration midwifery programme can be provided by a University, it must gain approval from the NMC. Approval means that the University programme complies with the standards set by the NMC in the document 'Standards for pre-registration midwifery education' (NMC 2009). The NMC approves the programme through an evaluation event where an expert midwife, who has been trained by the NMC to work on their behalf, scrutinises the documentation and talks to midwife academics about its content as well as current students and midwives in clinical practice. The expert midwife will then make a judgement about the suitability of the programme to support student midwives to be appropriately educated in order to take on the role as a registered midwife.

As well as the NMC requirements, midwifery education programmes must meet a variety of University standards including academic entry, assessment criteria and academic progression. The Quality Assurance Agency, a UK-wide body, also sets standards that enable an organisation to be called a University as well as more specific standards related to the academic level of programmes such as BSc (Hons), for example (QAAHE 2001). These requirements will also be confirmed at the same evaluation event that the NMC attends.

On-going monitoring of the quality of the programme in both practice and the University is undertaken annually by the NMC to ensure that the standards remain rooted in the programme and that they are maintained at a high level. Quality monitoring is also undertaken by the commissioners (the organisation(s) who pay the University to run the programme) such as the Department of Health (DH) in England, and equivalent in Northern Ireland, Scotland and Wales. The commissioners have organisations which work on their behalf and have a more hands-on approach to reviewing the programmes. Feedback is then reported upwards to give a national picture of what is happening.

The standards set by the NMC not only cover requirements during your programme but also before gaining a place to study midwifery. Your journey through the recruitment and selection progress would have been influenced by the University regulations and the standards set by the NMC. For example:

■ Midwifery clinicians should be directly involved in the interview process.

■ Applicants must provide evidence of literacy and numeracy of a satisfactory level to achieve the programme outcomes.

■ Applicants must demonstrate they have good health and good character sufficient for safe and effective practice.

Good health and good character are fundamental to the fitness to practice of a midwife (NMC 2010). Good character is based on an

> "Individual's conduct, behaviour and attitude. It takes into account any convictions, cautions and impending charges that are likely to be unsuitable with professional registration"
>
> (NMC 2010:8).

Good health in this context

> "Does not mean the absence of any disability or health condition. Many disabled people and those with health conditions are able to practise with or without adjustments to support their practice"
>
> NMC (2010:8).

It is strongly advised to declare any disability you may have on your application. This means that an early meeting with the University and relevant practice partners will be able to be arranged with you. The purpose of this is to discuss the requirements of the programme in an open and transparent way and determine whether reasonable adjustments may be required for either your practice placements or academic learning. Best practice indicates that the earlier this discussion takes place the easier reasonable adjustments can be implemented. (See Chapter 2 – section referred to as 'Support for you while in placement'). The NMC standards for midwifery education also outlines a number of guiding principles relating to professional competence and fitness for practice as well as the promotion and facilitation of the normal physiological process of childbirth. Competence is the ability to practise safely and effectively without the need for direct supervision. Students must demonstrate competence in a range of settings and many different scenarios during the antenatal, intrapartum and postnatal periods, as well as assessment and care of the newborn baby. Demonstration of competence must be supported by appropriate knowledge. The NMC states six key areas that you must demonstrate competence in at the point of registration (See Box 1.1) (NMC 2009:4):

The NMC and practice requirements

The NMC require a minimum of 50% of the programme to take place in practice, providing direct care to women, babies and their families. While in clinical practice you will be under the direct or indirect supervision of a midwife. Direct supervision means you will be working

---

Box 1.1 Six key areas of competence at point of registration

■ Sound, evidence-based knowledge of facilitating the physiology of childbirth and the newborn, and be competent in applying this in practice

■ Is knowledgeable of psychological, social, emotional and spiritual factors that may positively or adversely influence normal physiology, and be competent in applying this to practice

■ Appropriate interpersonal skills to support women and their families

■ Skills in managing obstetric and neonatal emergencies, underpinned by appropriate knowledge

■ Being autonomous practitioners and lead carers to women experiencing normal childbirth and being able to support women throughout their pregnancy, labour, birth and postnatal period, in all settings including midwife-led units, birthing centres and home

■ Being able to undertake critical decision making to support appropriate referral of either the woman or baby to other health professionals or agencies where there is recognition of normal processes being adversely affected or compromised

closely with a practising midwife, so they can directly observe what you are doing. As you become more skilled, independent and confident in your practise, the midwife may feel it more appropriate to supervise you indirectly. On these occasions, care has been delegated to you in a safe and responsible manner. Indirect supervision is more likely when you are in the later stages of your programme. The midwife, however, must be easily contactable and provide a level of support that is safe for both the women and yourself.

Standard 17 in the NMC 'Standards for pre registration midwifery education' (2009:21) gives examples of how the six key areas identified above can be achieved in practice using the following headings:

■ Effective midwifery practice

■ Professional and ethical practice

■ Developing the individual midwife and other

■ Achieving quality care through evaluation and research

Supporting each of the above are the Essential Skills Clusters (ESCs) given in Fig. 1.6.

The NMC views the ESCs as essential to your learning in practice and this is why they are specific requirements for you to achieve by the end of your programme.

The variety and length of practice placements may differ between universities. Often this depends on what placements are available in the local community and NHS Trusts as well and how many students are on the programme. For example some universities place student midwives in general medical and surgical wards where traditionally student nurses are placed (see Chapter 7 on 'Wider Experiences'). However, other universities prefer to demonstrate that the knowledge and skills gained in these placements can be met entirely in a midwifery setting. Despite the variety of environments there is still the need for student midwives to meet all the NMC requirements by the end of their programme.

The NMC and assessment of practice

Chapter 3 'Assessment of Practice' goes into depth about this important aspect of your practice placements. A brief explanation only is therefore included here. Since 2008 pre-registration midwifery programmes have needed to ensure that the assessment of direct hands-on practice is graded. This means that rather than just receiving a pass or fail judgement about your level of competence in practice, a system recognised by the University such as a percentage grade (50%, 60%, and 70%), or letter (A, B, C, and D) will be used to distinguish more clearly your level of practice. The grades awarded must contribute to the final outcome of the award. Universities use a variety of different practice assessment tools as the NMC does not stipulate one particular method that should be used (Fisher et al. 2015). Whatever

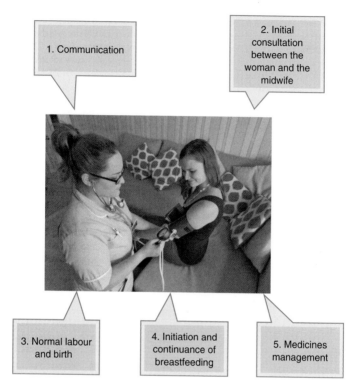

Figure 1.6 Essential skills clusters.

method is used in your University will have been agreed by the NMC at the curriculum approval event previously described. Some areas within the United Kingdom are seeking a similar practice assessment tool; in London for example a number of universities are in the process of agreeing a common tool in order to provide some consistency in how students are assessed in practice. This is particularly relevant as clinical areas may be shared by more than one University.

A range of people will be involved in assessing your practice. The NMC sets the standards for those midwives who support learning and make judgements about your ability to practise

(NMC 2008), who are known as sign-off mentors. Chapter 3 goes into more detail about their role. Others such as a member of the midwifery teaching team and the women you care for may also be asked to contribute in various ways. The NMC advises that midwife teachers should spend approximately 20% of the normal teaching hours assisting in the support of learning in practice. Each University will have a particular way that this is achieved and how you can make contact with them when they are in the clinical area.

Raising concerns

The new NMC Code published in March 2015, has meant the NMC Document 'Guidance on professional conduct for nursing and midwifery students' (2011) has been withdrawn. This is because the content within the 2011 publication for student nurses and midwives has now been incorporated within the Code (2015). The Code is therefore central to your practice as a student midwife and will continue to be during your midwifery career. The pre-registration programme you will be following will enable you to use these standards demonstrating your commitment to upholding them. The Code (2015) is based on four themes that nurses and midwives are expected to adhere to

- prioritise people,

- practise effectively,

- preserve safety and

- promote professionalism and trust.

Poor standards of care in the NHS and other health care organisations often attracts media attention such as that at Mid Staffordshire which culminated in the 'Report of the Mid Staffordshire NHS Foundation Trust Public Inquiry', chaired by Robert Francis QC (Francis 2013). Although this has been mostly related to nursing and medical care, reports of care in midwifery that has fallen below an acceptable standard have also been published (Care Quality Commission – CQC 2013; NMC 2014). You may be in the unfortunate position to witness poor care and are unsure what to do about it. You have a duty to put the interests of people in your care first and act to protect them if you consider they may be at risk. The NMC provides guidance for all nurses, midwives and pre-registration nursing and midwifery students about how to do this (NMC 2013).

It might not be easy for you to raise a concern but there are people you can go to for advice and support. All Universities should have a policy available to students about how to raise concerns and it is important you know where to find the document and what it says. Generally the advice would be to inform your mentor or academic tutor as soon as you believe that you, a colleague or anyone else may be putting someone at risk. If you believe that harm has already been suffered, then you must let a qualified health professional know immediately. If someone tells you they are not happy with their care, then you should seek help from your mentor or academic advisor/personal tutor. A hypothetical example is provided by the

NMC on raising concerns: http://www
.nmc-uk.org/Nurses-and-midwives/
Raising-and-escalating-concerns/
Toolkit/case-studies/. After reading the
case study read page 4 of the NMC
document, Raising concerns: guidance
for nurses and midwives (NMC 2013).
Referring to the section 'Your role in
raising concerns' make notes about
whether you think the student acted
appropriately and why. Next, read the
4 themes that the Code is based on.
Which themes do you think the case
study is referring to and why?

Guidance on using social media and social networking as a student

Luisa Cescutti-Butler

The rise in the use of social media has
soared over the last 10 years, with Facebook and Twitter being the most popular. The NMC in its document
"Facebook trials and tribulations: Social
networking sites and their joys and dangers" says of the 25, 789, 200 users of
Facebook that 77, 580 listed their occu-
pation as nurse, midwife or health visitor
(Facebook, 2011a cited in Jaeger 2011).
Chances are that you yourself use one or
more of the numerous social media
applications which are easily accessible
via your personal smart phone or tablet
to connect with friends and family. Many
midwives and student midwives are
doing likewise, enabling them to link
professionally with colleagues to share

ideas and resources or to network
through an online community (Byrom &
Byrom 2014). One of the advantages of
social media is everybody has a voice and
you can communicate with people who
would otherwise be inaccessible to you
(Byrom & Byrom 2014). Examples
include linking up with student midwives
from other universities, connecting with
key midwifery professionals and joining
in with health and social care discussions
on Twitter. Jane Cummings (NHS
England Chief Nursing Officer) and
Cathy Warwick (Chief Executive of
the RCM) are two of the senior leaders
who see the benefits of social media and
regularly use it as an opportunity to reach
as many people as possible (Chinn &
Foord 2014). In addition service-users
of maternity care (mothers/fathers/
partners) are using platforms such as
Facebook and Twitter to share their
experiences, connect with healthcare
professionals and importantly, campaign
for change (Byrom & Byrom 2014)

It appears, however, that many student midwives are wary of using social
media in case they do something 'wrong',
but if you follow the guidelines as set out
by your professional 'Code' (NMC
2015) and your University, you should
keep yourself safe. The NMC supports
the use of social media, as do many
senior leaders within the NHS (Chinn &
Foord 2014). Don't be afraid of using it
providing you follow the 'guidelines'.
Find out what your University's policy
is on using social media – read and
absorb its contents. While bearing
these in mind, the following 6 Ps should
also help you consider what is appropriate or not.

1 Professional.

As a student midwife you must act professionally at all times. What happens on your social media pages in a personal capacity can still reflect upon you as a student.

2 Positive.

Be positive when posting on social media. Don't complain about your busy shift or the lazy midwife you may have worked with. Don't re-post any posts which may be deemed offensive; you will still be linked to them. If you are tagged in any inappropriate messages etc, remove the links, un-tag yourself and if applicable report the content to the relevant authorities.

3 Person/woman, patient free.

You must keep posts person/ women & patient free. Do not discuss on any site how you facilitated a wonderful birth. Never accept a 'friend request' from a woman whose birth you have facilitated. Do not post any pictures of women who are service users.

4 Protect yourself.

Protect your professionalism, your reputation and yourself. It may be difficult to have separate accounts; one for you as a professional and one for your personal life. To make life simple, have one account and use it wisely but remember to uphold your profession.

5 Privacy.

Check your privacy settings & respect the privacy of others. Use robust passwords and change them regularly. Avoid using the same password for all your online interactions. Avoid the common passwords, for example your date of birth (DOB), or your child's name and DOB etc.

6 Pause before you post.

Always THINK before you post anything. Once it's on, it's there for the whole world to see. THINK: would you want your post to be seen by your family, your personal tutor, your mentors or the Head of Midwifery? If in doubt, do not post. Also, don't post in anger or quickly.

(Nursing and Midwifery Board of Ireland 2013)

#Wecommunities available on http://www.wenurses.co.uk/ has a variety of resources (articles and presentations) on how to use social media safely. Much of the information has been written for nurses (students and qualified), but is equally applicable to you as a student midwife. Chinn & Foord (2014) have written a short article busting the myths around Twitter usage which is a useful read.

Social media can also help midwifery tutors to effectively connect with students. In most universities, traditional methods of communication are used with students, the most popular being email. Often, if a response is required, it can take several days especially if the student is busy in placement. The solution was to try Facebook. I created a group page which is only open to midwifery students who are clinically based in the NHS Trust to which I link. First-year students are added as soon as they are officially enrolled at University, and third-year students are taken off once they have qualified. Guidelines have been set which have been respected by all the students using it. As a medium

Luisa Cescutti-Butler
1 July · Edited

UPTODATE:
- is provided for you by the Healthcare Library.
- answers your clinical queries quickly.
- saves you time.
- ensures your patients get the best evidence-based care.
- is highly rated by practicing clinicians like yourselves.
- Access directly from the Trust Intranet or click on the link – no password required on site.

Want to know more? Drop in to the Healthcare Library on Friday 11th July, 12pm – 3pm, or contact library.office@xxxxxx.nhs.uk to arrange a 1:1 or department visit.

Like · Comment

✓ Seen by 24

for communication, it works very well with students responding to requests much quicker than the traditional email. An extract presented above highlights how the page is used to communicate with students.

The students, however, find value in the Facebook group themselves. Many of their postings relate to shift patterns and whether the off-duty is out. Students are free to post any interesting articles/links that others may find interesting. See below for examples of how students use the page.

When students were asked whether they felt the Facebook group page served their needs the following quotes demonstrate some of their views:

"I like this group as it does make communicating easier especially with other years as I wouldn't really know them otherwise and it's nice to be able to ask questions and get a response from people who have been through the same things"

First-year student.

"I love all your articles along with being able to communicate with peeps as necessary"

Third-year student.

"I agree. It's great to be able to keep in touch and it's really nice when it's across all three years too as we might not have been able to communicate as much being on placement at different times etc"

Second-year student.

"Hi Luisa, I've found it really helpful and good to have for communication with you and other years when needed, it's almost guaranteed to get a quick response which is great. And love the articles x"

Second-year student.

As can be seen, students seem to value the Facebook group page. From my perspective I usually get a response to a query fairly quickly. Most of all the students really like being able to get to know each other – especially those from different years – and to ask questions or for advice about their practice area in a safe environment.

Extract 1

Hey all, Just asked my community midwife to confirm what drugs we carry for home births and she said:

-2 Ampoules Syntometrine
-2 Ampoules Ergometrine
-2 Ampoules Lignocaine
-Paracetomol
-2 Ampoules of Vitamin K
-Cylinder of Entonox

Hopefully this can help you with emergency skills and anything else and hopefully its correct, let me know if you think it anything different 😄 xx

Extract 2

Hi guys! lovely to see u all today. I thought I would compile a list of things that would be useful for (future) first years to know how to do. As many students may not have been in a hospital or care environment. These are some of my thoughts as they are things that can be shown to them prior to commencing placement:
1. How to wash a woman and provide personal care. 2. How to thoroughly clean a labour room or postnatal bed space using the correct stuff. 3. Catheter care, How to empty one without spilling 😄, where it goes etc. 4. How to af feed babies (may sound silly) but those that have never done it may find it difficult. ie when to wind, best position to hold them in. And it may be something you have to do early on in practice.
I cant think of anything else right now. What do u guys think? 😄

Extract 3

Are the shifts for week beginning 21 Jul up? Thanks in advance 😄

Like Comment

✔ Seen by 24

To conclude, using social media has many benefits providing you understand the boundaries. Try it and see. There are many advantages and as a medium it can help enhance your learning and connect you with people far and wide. #WeMidwives at @WeMidwives (part of the @WeNurses community) on Twitter, supports and connects the tweeting Midwives Community. It is a great forum to link up with midwifery students and key midwifery professionals (and others, such as obstetricians) both in the United Kingdom and internationally.

Conclusion

This chapter has highlighted the processes you need to go through to qualify as a midwife including outlining the rules and regulations that govern your practice. First you are expected to successfully complete an approved midwifery education programme, following which you are then required to register with the NMC which provides you with a license to practise. This license, including an annual fee, requires renewing each year and you will have to prove to the NMC that you remain competent to practise as a midwife, have submitted your annual Intention to Practise form (required at the time of writing) and remain updated in order to provide safe and effective care. In addition, the chapter has explored aspects of midwifery care including the use of language, the 6Cs, and humanisation of care. By considering how you can incorporate these elements into your daily midwifery practice will ensure you truly provide woman and family centred care and be the midwife that is 'with woman!' Finally the chapter concludes around a discussion on the advantages of social media and how you as a student can safely use it to enhance your learning, make useful connections and contribute to midwifery care and practice.

Text box 1: Please see vignette 1.2 'Meeting Suzy where student midwife Millie has incorporated aspects of the 6Cs and humanisation of care into her practice.

Vignette 1.2   A reflection on meeting Suzy

Suzy was the first mother I met in my student midwifery training, on placement in the community. Her story was compelling and it stirred up a lot of emotion for me. This reflection uses Borton's (1970) reflective model to explore the psychology behind Suzy's situation, and the impact her situation had on me. All names have been changed in accordance with the NMC code of conduct (2008).

On my first shift, my mentor and I visited Suzy and her new baby Esme for their day 5 postnatal check. My mentor gave me Suzy's background beforehand: that she was a 17-year-old woman who had conceived her child with her stepfather, whom she had known since she was 6 years old. Social services (Child Protection) were involved regarding Esme's welfare, including the possibility of her being groomed by Suzy's stepfather. I was shocked – the first woman I was going to meet was in such a vulnerable, difficult situation, and I immediately visualised a dysfunctional and inadequate teenager. Not only would I have to observe and digest the entire postnatal check, but also in what I thought would be rather difficult circumstances [. . .] and it made me feel incredibly nervous and worried.

We arrived at Suzy's foster accommodation where my mentor and I were met at the door by a shy- and sweet-looking woman, holding Esme close to her chest. We chatted to her first about her situation. I was amazed at how besotted with love she was for her baby, and realised that I had earlier prejudged her. We learnt that she felt very lonely, because her mother did not visit, and her foster family were out working most of the time. She was not allowed contact with her stepfather, and she planned to move north to live with her biological father. Before Social Services became involved she had hoped to go to France to live with her stepfather, and her mother (who was apparently happy with the situation).

My mentor performed the postnatal check whilst I observed. Suzy picked up Esme afterwards to breastfeed her. Suzy was so young, and I saw her as needing nurturing and support herself, but now she was comfortable and competent, performing the most natural act as if it was the best thing in the world for her.

[. . .] As the week progressed I felt that a trusting relationship formed between Suzy, my mentor and me. Suzy expressed her anger at being restricted from seeing her stepfather, seemingly unaware of the potential dangers to her baby. When the legalities around safeguarding Esme were explained again Suzy became angry as she was desperate for her partner to meet his new daughter. I felt saddened by how naïve she seemed, then I remembered how vulnerable I had felt at that age, how everything could be so confusing; how on earth could she manage to nurture a newborn without anyone there for her? But Suzy seemed to be coping, and to be strongly bonded to her baby. We [. . .] explained everything again clearly and calmly. She was aware that if she made contact with her stepfather, Esme would be removed by Social Services. This brought tears to her eyes and I truly felt, at the time, that there was nothing on this earth that would risk her losing her daughter.

I learnt the following week from my mentor that Suzy had visited her stepfather and that the police had been called by a neighbour. [. . .] I felt shattered by this, and confused. How could Suzy? She had appeared to love Esme with all her heart. I could not bear to think of her without her baby.

I was initially shocked by Suzy's fluctuating behaviour between anger, infatuation for Esme, confusion, and impulsive decision making. On later reflection, emotional isolation for any new mother with responsibility for a new life, even without Suzy's additional problems, would be unbearable. Suzy needed love and support herself and the only person she saw who could give it was her stepfather. She was also under the influence of hormonal changes associated with the postnatal period, such as progesterone withdrawal and prolactin release, which activate nurturing behaviour towards the newborn, but can alter the mother's emotional state, which may lead to depressive disorders (Brunton & Russell 2008).

Suzy's age was a major influence as well. Being an adolescent, she was experiencing an already difficult period of vulnerability, adjustment and brain development (Steinberg 2005). She was subject to heightened emotional

(continued)

reactivity resulting from social interactions with the people that she knew (Casey et al. 2008). Although she was probably aware that the rational decision would be to cut off contact with her stepfather, her age may have caused her limbic system – her emotional powers – to take control, therefore relying less on intellectual capability, resulting in taking a huge risk when deciding to visit her stepfather (Casey et al. 2008). It is also possible that Suzy's need for nurturing and support for herself from the man she loved and who was the father of her baby, outweighed the risk of losing the baby.

I have learnt that it is of the upmost importance to gain extra professional support when dealing with adolescents; women who themselves still need mothering, and are experiencing the self-definition process (Raphael-Leff 2005). Whether we are aware of them or not, we all make classifications and judgements about people based on experience, stereotyping and word of mouth (Paradice 2002). A judgemental attitude by healthcare professionals can have negative consequences and influence a woman's behaviour, and it is important to practise both self and inter-personal awareness (Paradice 2002).

I feel that I learnt one of the most valuable lessons in my first week from meeting Suzy; that is, to treat every woman as an individual. Our preconceived ideas can often be proved wrong, as when I initially prejudged Suzy by stereotype. Additionally, when I was shocked by Suzy being 'naive' and then 'willing' to take the risk of losing the baby she appeared to love and want, I was not truly empathising with her particular – and tragically conflictual circumstances. Best practice is to be open minded and non-judgemental, which I believe to be fundamental qualities to pursue a career in midwifery.

References

Borton T (1970) *Reach, Touch and Teach*. McGraw-Hill Book Company, New York.

Brunton PJ, Russell JA (2008) The expectant brain: adapting for motherhood. *Nat Rev, Neuroscience* 9: 11–25.

Casey BJ, Jones RM, Hare TA (2008) The adolescent brain. *Ann New York Acad Sci* 1124: 111–126.

Nursing and Midwifery Council (2008) *The Code: Standards of Conduct, Performance and Ethics for Nurses and Midwives*. Nursing and Midwifery Council, London.

Paradice R (2002) *Psychology for Midwives*. Quay Books, Wiltshire.

Raphael-Leff J (2005) *Psychological Processes of Childbearing*. The Anna Freud Centre, Great Britain.

Steinberg L (2005) Cognitive and affective development in adolescence. *TRENDS Cogn Sci* 9(2): 69–74.

Millie Westwood
Third-year midwifery student, Bournemouth University, Dorset, UK
Reproduced with permission of Millie Westwood.

References

Association for Improvements in the Maternity Services (AIMS) (2012) Top ten tips for what women want from their midwives. *Essent MIDIRS* 3: 27–31.

Bryar R (1991) Research and Individualised Care in Midwifery. In: Robinson S and Thomson A (eds). *Midwives, Research and Childbirth*. II, 48–71, Chapman Hall, London.

Byrom S (2013) *Childbirth and the language we use: does it really matter*. Available at http://sheenabyrom.com/2013/04/12/childbirth-and-the-language-we-use-does-it-really-matter/ (last accessed 01 July 2014).

Byrom S, Byrom A (2014) Social media: connecting women and midwives globally. *MIDIRS Midwifery Digest* 24: 141–149.

Carboon F (1999) Language power and change. *ACMI J* 12 (4): 19–22.

Chinn T, Foord D (2014) *Celebrities and Trolls . . . the many myths of Twitter for nurses . . . busted!* Available at http://www.nhsemployers.org (last accessed 20 August 2014).

Care Quality Commission (CQC) (2013) *National Survey from the 2013 survey of women's experiences of maternity care*. http://www.cqc.org.uk/content/maternity-services-survey-2013 (last accessed 29 July 2014).

Department of Health (1993) *Changing Childbirth Part 1: Report of the Expert Maternity Group*. DoH, London.

Department of Health (2007) *Maternity Matters: Choice, Access and Continuity of Care in a Safe Service*. DoH, London.

Department of Health (2009) *Delivering High Quality Midwifery Care: The Priorities, Opportunities and Challenges for Midwives*. DoH, London.

Department of Health (2010) *Midwifery 2020: Delivering expectations Midwifery 2020*. Cambridge, Programme Board.

Department of Health (2012). *Liberating the NHS: No Decision About Me, Without Me – Government Response to the Consultation*. DoH, London.

European Parliament (2013) *Recognition of professional qualifications*. Available at http://ec.europa.eu/internal_market/qualifications/policy_developments/legislation/index_en.htm (last accessed 29 July 2014).

Fisher M, Bower H, Chenery-Morris S, Jackson J, Way S (2015) *A scoping study to explore the application and impact of grading practice in pre-registration midwifery programmes across the united kingdom*. Nurse Education in Practice [under review].

Flint C (1986) *Sensitive Midwifery*. Heinemann Midwifery, London.

Francis R (2013) *The Mid Staffordshire: Report of the Mid Staffordshire NHS Foundation Trust Public Enquiry*. The Stationary Office, London.

Furber CM, Thomson AM (2010) The power of language: a secondary analysis of a qualitative study exploring English midwives' support of mother's baby-feeding practice. *Midwifery* 26: 232–240.

Garcia J (1982) Women's views of antenatal care. In: Enkin M and Chalmers I (eds), *Effectiveness and Satisfaction in Antenatal Care*, 81, 81–91. The Lavenham Press Limited, Suffolk.

Hunter L (2006) Women give birth and pizzas are delivered: language and western childbirth paradigms. *J Midwifery & Women's Health* 51: 119–124.

International Confederation of Midwives (2011) *ICM Definition of a Midwife*. Available at http://www.internationalmidwives.org/assets/uploads/documents/Definition%20of%20the%20Midwife%20-%202011.pdf (last accessed 9 September 2014).

Ireland J, van Teijlingen E (2013) Normal birth: social-medical model. *The Practising Midwife* 61 (12): 17–20.

Jaeger A (2011) *Facebook trials and tribulations: Social networking sites and their joys and dangers*. Available at http://www.nmc-uk.org (last accessed 1 July 2014).

Lewis P (2014) Professional indemnity insurance – the making or breaking of midwifery. *Br J Midwifery* 22 (11): 766.

Lichtman R (2013) Midwives don't deliver or catch: a humble vocabulary suggestion. *J Midwifery & Women's Health* 124–125.

NHS Commissioning Board (2012) *Compassion in Practice – our culture of compassionate care*. Available at http://www.england.nhs.uk/nursingvision/ (last accessed 9 September 2014).

Nursing and Midwifery Council (2008) *Standards to Support Learning and Assessment in Practice*. NMC, London.

Nursing and Midwifery Council (2009) *Standards for Pre-registration Midwifery Education*. NMC, London.

Nursing and Midwifery Council (2009) *Guidance on professional conduct for nursing and midwifery students*. Available at http://www.nmc-uk.org (last accessed 18 August 2014).

Nursing and Midwifery Council (2010) *Good health and good character: Guidance for approved educations institutions*. Available at http://www.nmc-uk.org/Documents/Guidance/nmcGood-HealthAndGoodCharacterGuidanceForApprovedEducationInstitutions.PDF (last accessed 29 July 2014).

Nursing and Midwifery Council (2011) *Guidance on Professional Conduct for Nursing and Midwifery Students*. NMC, London.

Nursing and Midwifery Council (2012) *The Midwives Rules and Standards*. NMC, London.

Nursing and Midwifery Council (2013) *Raising Concerns: Guidance for Nurses and Midwives*. NMC, London.

Nursing and Midwifery Council (2014) *Extraordinary LSA Review: Princess Elizabeth Hospital, Health and Social Services Department, Guernsey*. NMC, London.

Nursing and Midwifery Council (2015) *The Code: Standards of Conduct, Performance and Ethics for Nurses and Midwives*. NMC, London.

Nursing and Midwifery Board of Ireland (NMBI) (2013) *Guidance to Nurses and Midwives on Social Media and Social Networking*. Available at http://www.nmbi.ie (last accessed 1 July 2014).

Pollard K (2011) How midwives' discursive practices contribute to the maintenance of the status quo in English maternity care. *Midwifery* 27: 612–619.

Prochaska E (2013) The importance of dignity in childbirth. *Br J Midwifery* 21: 82.

Quality Assurance Agency for Higher Education (2001) *Subject Benchmark Statement: Health Care Programmes*. Available at http://www.qaa.ac.uk (last accessed 9 September 2014).

Renfrew M, McFadden A, Bastos MH, Campbell J, Channon AA, Cheung NF, Silva AD, Downe S, Kennedy HP, Malata A, McCormick F, Wick L, Declercq E (2014) *Midwifery and quality care: findings from a new evidence-informed framework for maternal and newborn care*. Available at http://ac.els-cdn.com/S0140673614607893/1-s2.0-S0140673614607893-main.pdf?_tid=774ce6ee-29e8-11e4-9ecc-00000aab0f01&acdnat=1408704093_5ca70e2ad13fc8d398d1ed67c5d22cbc (last accessed 22 August 2014).

Robertson A (1999) *Watch your language*. Available at https://www.birthinternational.com/articles/childbirth-education/29-watch-your-language (last accessed 1 July 2014).

Romney ML, Gordon H (1981) Is your enema really necessary? *Br Med J* 282: 1269–1271.

Royal College of Midwives (1997) *Normality in midwifery*. Royal College of Midwives, London.

Simkin P, Stewart M, Shearer B, Glantz JC, Rooks J, Lyerly A, Chalmers B, Keirse M (2012) Roundtable discussion: the language of birth. *Birth* 39: 156–164.

The Maternity Services Action Group (2011) *A Refreshed Framework for Maternity Care in Scotland*. Scottish Government, Edinburgh.

Thomas BG (2003) The Disempowering Concept of Risk. In *Midwifery Best Practice*. (ed. S. Wickham) pp. 3–5. Books for Midwives, London.

Thompson AM (1980) Planned or unplanned? Are midwives ready for the 1980s? *Midwives Chron Nurs Notes* 93: 68–72.

Todres L, Galvin, G, Holloway I (2009) The humanising of healthcare: a value framework for qualitative research. *Int J Qualit Stud Health Well-being* 4 (3): 68–77.

van Teijlingen E (2005) A critical analysis of the medical model as used in the study of pregnancy and childbirth. *Sociol Res Online* 10. www.socresonline.org.uk/10/2/teijlingen.html (last accessed 9 September 2014).

Walsh D, El-Nemer A, Downe S (2004) Risk, Safety and the Study of Physiological Birth. In *Normal Childbirth: Evidence and Debate*. (ed. S. Downe) pp. 103–120. Churchill Livingstone, London.

Further resources

Feminist Midwife Blog: Room seven delivered, no complications. http://www.feministmidwife.com/2014/07/10/room-seven-delivered-no-complications/.

Natalie Boxall discusses how the use of social media can benefit midwives by making connections and sharing experiences. Available: https://www.rcm.org.uk/content/social-awareness.

Chapter 2
PREPARATION FOR PRACTICE

Henrietta Otley

Introduction

Most midwifery courses are divided equally between time spent studying theory in University and practical placements outside in a variety of practice settings. These placements usually start early on in your course and are your opportunity to learn essential skills on the job.

Spending shifts on delivery suite, in midwife-led units, at antenatal clinics or attending homebirths with the community midwives, learning patient care skills in the gynaecology ward or somewhere else you may be sent is really exciting and probably just what you've joined the midwifery course to do. It can also be quite intimidating.

This chapter will address the important things you need to know and do in order to be prepared for practice in a clinical setting. You will find more specific information in other chapters. It will advise on time management, working with a variety of mentors, striking a good work–life balance, coping with night shifts, working alongside professionals from other disciplines and getting to grips with the culture of the NHS. To help you make the most of the exciting opportunities coming your way and guide you through the intermittently calm and choppy waters of your years as a student midwife, this chapter includes top tips for thriving out in practice, a glossary to demystify the midwifery and obstetric language you're going to come across and an introduction to the sources of support and information that are out there.

The theory–practice gap

In order to promote best practice and constantly improve midwifery services, your University should teach you midwifery ideals. However, you may sometimes find that when you are out on the wards with your mentor, the realities you see are not always the exemplary practices you had expected (Barkley 2011). This 'theory–practice gap' can be a bit of a shock.

The Hands-on Guide to Midwifery Placements, First Edition.
Edited by Luisa Cescutti-Butler and Margaret Fisher.
© 2016 John Wiley & Sons, Ltd. Published 2016 by John Wiley & Sons, Ltd.

If you have come into midwifery to make a difference, keep in mind the way you want to practice and learn from your mentors' best habits. Even if you sometimes feel powerless to change things, remember that, as a midwife of the future, your experience on placement and your learning process are very important. You may feel like a small cog in the machinery of the large hospital you find yourself in, but the support you are giving the woman you are with will be of great significance to her.

The NHS has a particular culture, and midwifery culture has its own quirks. Getting to grips with these while still remaining true to your aims of providing quality care to childbearing women and their families means that your first year of training can be the most challenging. This transition can be particularly difficult for students who are already registered nurses, as adapting to the different culture and context of care of midwifery along with the increased expectations of this autonomous profession may prove testing. It's important to acknowledge that adapting, or at least coming to terms with new ways of working and thinking, can be difficult and isn't for everyone. Make the most of any opportunity you have to talk to second- and third-year midwifery students who should be able to reassure you that seemingly insurmountable concerns will become quite manageable over time.

Work–life balance

Maybe you have run a business, held a high-powered job or managed a demanding family. Doubtless you have accumulated worthwhile skills for keeping on top of your busy life. As a student midwife, you will need to reach a whole new level of efficiency to enable you to contribute to being part of a team on a hectic delivery suite, caring for eight postnatal women and babies with complex needs, running a packed antenatal clinic with 15 minute appointments, being poised to react appropriately to emergencies and so on. But don't worry, while it may initially be alarming, you have the 3 years of your course to develop the skills you'll need. Those who have practised as nurses will be one step ahead in that you will have already learned to juggle and multi-task in your professional role. You will also already be familiar with many of the aspects discussed below.

Unlike many University courses, with midwifery you're not looking at long, lazy summer holidays or really very much down time at all. Apart from a few brief weeks each year, the rule tends to be that if you're not on placement, you are in University and any other time is spent in private study. It is very common for student midwives to have young children and many find it a tricky balancing act to carry on being a good parent and keep on top of the demands of the course. It may take a good few months to determine how this will best work for you and your family, and, as you will soon be advising new mothers postnatally, take all the help you are offered. Many student midwives start the course with a part time job; however, most find that they are not able to sustain this double life because the course absorbs all their time and vitality (Lee & Busby 2010).

However you choose to manage things, you're going to need to be very organised, to make some decisions and to find the right level for you. Is your priority to excel academically or to carry on being a good party host/run the school cake sales or whatever it is that you have been throwing your energy into up to now? Once you qualify, you really will get your life back, but midwifery training can be all-consuming.

Your University will probably give you a uniform to wear while on placements. While it can be wonderful to put this outfit on and step into the identity of a student midwife, in the eyes of others around you in a busy hospital it will also define you and depersonalise you (Fig. 2.1). A social science lecturer turned student midwife sums up how disempowering this transformation can feel:

'A confident, professional woman before I began my training, once I put on my student uniform and became a novice at the bottom of a hierarchical structure, all my confidence, previous knowledge and life experience disappeared.'

Bosanquet (2002)

Fitting in, to some degree, is necessary and desirable, but try never to forget who you are, what you know and what you believe in. After all, midwifery training is supposed to turn you into a thoughtful, empathetic, capable midwife not an automaton.

Shift work

Wherever your placement is, you will notice the midwives poring over a much-used folder confusingly marked 'Off Duty'. This shows the shifts each midwife is to work for the month, and student midwives may be given – or asked to nominate – times to be on placement in the 'off duty' too. Your University will communicate with the midwifery coordinators about how many hours you are expected to attend and they should aim to ensure you work with your allocated mentor(s) as much as possible. At least 40% (two shifts) of your time must be spent being supervised (directly or indirectly) by your mentor and having this continuity helps you to get your skills and competencies signed off in your practice document.

Your shifts need to be documented on the off-duty along with the name of

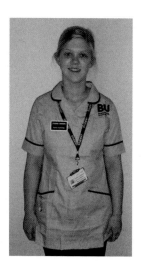

Figure 2.1 An example of a student midwife's uniform.

the midwife supervising you. It is essential that you always work under the direct or indirect supervision of a named midwife (or nurse). It is also important that your presence on a shift is recorded in case any follow-up is needed of staff and students, for example following a difficult incident. Some universities will require you to get each shift signed by the professional supporting you and this may be on your portfolio of evidence document.

While you are still training, you may be spared the full quota of shifts outside the normal 9-5, Monday to Friday that most people work. You will still have to get to grips with (and even embrace) the concept of a 24 hour service that might need you to be alert and effective at any time of day or night, any day of the week.

Healthcare Trusts differ, but normal shift options include a long day shift (up to 12 hours), shorter 'early' or 'late' shifts (around 7.5 hours) and night shifts which are usually between 10 and 12 hours. You can find out the timings of shifts by speaking to the University lecturer who liaises with your particular placement setting, with a second- or third-year student or by ringing up the unit you will be attending.

When you are in a stimulating environment and learning lots of new skills, it may initially be tiring working the long shifts. Bring lots of snacks to get you through the shift and try to pace yourself – you have a lot of time to learn what you need to, you don't have to understand it all at once. Remember to drink lots because you'll get much more tired if you are dehydrated. Try to take your

breaks with your mentor, then you can sit in the staff room and debrief by discussing what you've experienced if you need to. Particularly at the beginning of your training, you should not be left 'babysitting' a situation while your mentor takes her break. You also need a certain amount of flexibility when negotiating your breaks. For example if you are looking after a woman during advanced labour, it would not be appropriate to leave her because it's your lunch time! On other occasions, the woman you are caseloading (see Chapter 6) may be on delivery suite in early labour when you are called in to care for her. As each woman's labour is individual in its length, you may be with her all day and even long into the evening. It is important you recognise that if you don't have a break (it is illegal according to the European Working Time Directive to work 12 hours or more without a break), being tired impacts on your performance and your concentration. If your mentor does not facilitate a break for you (you are entitled to two 20 minute breaks if you are working a 12 hour shift), it is your responsibility to voice your concerns to the shift co-ordinator.

Night shifts

If you have worked nights before or enjoy a dynamic social life which keeps you up till the early hours or if your young children have got you practiced in functioning adequately at unsociable times, then night shifts may not pose a great challenge for you. If you find the idea of them daunting, be reassured that there are things you can do to make them manageable. For midwives, night shifts are a fact of life.

It is understandable that you might want to shy away from night shifts at first, but if that is when your mentor is working, then you will need to spend time together. The atmosphere and pace on a night shift can be very different from the day shift and is worth experiencing. The advantages of working at night include greater autonomy for the midwives as the doctors are often asleep. There tends to be a rather calmer atmosphere without the bustle and stress of clinics, consultants' rounds, ward attenders and visitors. If you want to increase the number of births you attend, then nights will provide you with that opportunity – more women give birth at night and there will be fewer students around competing with you to catch their babies. With the right approach, night shifts are quite manageable and can be rather magical.

People who do lots of long haul travel soon work out that a combination of planning wisely but not overthinking the situation is the best preparation for adjusting to being awake at unfamiliar times and coping with interrupted circadian rhythms. Lots of research has been done into effective shift work, much of it in a hospital setting because of the serious potential effects of staff fatigue and delayed responses on patient safety (HSE 2006).

As you get accustomed to night shifts, you will probably find a routine that works for you. You must emphatically defend your sleep, telling those around you when you should not be disturbed. If you have young children at home, you will need to get someone else to take care of them quietly – cat napping while looking after them will leave you exhausted.

Prepare the room you will sleep in carefully. Because light is a particularly powerful factor in resetting your body clock, the room must be dark and you may well need an eye mask and ear plugs. Get rid of all disturbances (TV, computer etc.) and turn your phone off. During the afternoon before the first night you work, give yourself time to relax by reading or listening to music and then try to get an hour or two of sleep. You may be surprised at how well this will sustain you throughout the night. Between night shifts you should aim for 6–8 hours of sleep, but after the last night allow yourself only 3 or 4 hours' sleep – you may find you stagger through the day a bit but it will mean you can go to bed at a normal time and reset your circadian rhythms for the next day.

Be aware of local policies around sleeping on night duty breaks in your own Trust as it may or may not be permitted. In order to stay alert during the night, you can eat light, healthy meals and drink plenty of fluid. Many midwives find that tea and coffee helps, but avoid caffeine towards the end of your shift. If you are feeling sleepy – you may struggle at around four or five in the morning – try to make yourself move around and expose yourself to bright lighting. It is best to avoid working more than three nights in a row.

Some midwives love night shifts and request to do as many of them as possible (working antisocial hours is paid extra), others try to avoid them. While you make your decision about how you feel about nights, try to approach them without fear. They may well be less disruptive and more manageable than you anticipate. Clearly, it is not advisable to work a night shift before a University day; many institutions will have a policy which recommends you do not attend a full day of lectures prior to or straight after a night shift.

Time management

Midwives are usually pretty busy, and the organisational skills required in the most exacting of settings on the postnatal ward or delivery suite of a large hospital can be quite remarkable. Do not worry, you are 'supernumerary' – this means you are not counted in the staffing levels – and should not be expected to pull any weight. It also enables you to be available to access a range of learning opportunities in other settings or shadowing staff (see Chapter 7 on Wider Midwifery Placements). You also have 3 years to become this efficient and your mentor(s) should provide plenty of guidance to help you manage your workload effectively and emerge satisfied – if exhausted – at the end of the shift.

Find out in advance what time your shift starts and finishes and leave plenty of time to travel, change into your uniform, make yourself a cup of tea, find a space in the fridge for your lunch and whatever else needs to happen before you're ready to begin.

Many midwives find it essential to write things down as they go along. At handover at the start of a shift on the postnatal ward, you will have a sheet listing every woman (and her baby) present and you will need to have quick access to information about her medical and social history, needs, drug regime and so on. You and your mentor will be allocated a particular section of the ward to look after; however, you may also have to answer call bells for other women, so you need to know something about everyone. For example, if a woman has called for breastfeeding support, the fact that she is a first time mum who has had a caesarean section will inform the care you offer her. Similarly, if you have noted down that she has a prosthetic left arm, you can spare her and yourself considerable awkwardness by taking a blood pressure reading on her right arm.

The postnatal ward tends to be the environment where keeping on top of what needs doing is most challenging. You may want to make an hour-by-hour plan of who needs what when – despite your best intentions and unless your organisational powers are extraordinary, you will need written prompts. Volunteer to help with the drugs round and you can briefly step out of a normal frenzied, multi-tasking environment where new demands seem constantly to take you away from achieving what is needed and into a focused job where everyone knows you mustn't be disturbed (it even says so on the tabard you may have to wear).

When you and your mentor take over one-to-one care of a woman in labour on delivery suite, it can be helpful to jot down the important things you need to remember on a scrap of paper as the information is given. Not only is it useful to be clear in your own mind about what is going on but it is also always fun as a student midwife to astonish the consultants on their ward round with a comprehensive list of a woman's medical history, drug regime, recent observations and progress.

You will have a long list of competencies you need to achieve; however, flexibility is essential in midwifery – it's always impressive to see a group of community midwives allocate the day's emerging workload. The unpredictability of how a midwifery shift will unfold makes it dynamic and exciting. While the day might not be turning out as you had anticipated, other opportunities will doubtless present themselves instead.

Working with mentors

If you have set your heart on becoming a midwife, there's a good chance that you may have an idealised perception of the people who make up the profession you want to enter. Many midwives are of course truly wonderful but the midwifery world, just like the wider population, is made up of all sorts of people. Some of them you'll get on with easily and some you won't. But midwifery mentoring isn't about making friends, it is a crucial part of educating midwives of the future – you – and it is part of every midwife's role. Usually within a year or two of qualifying, midwives are encouraged by their hospital Trust to complete a University module which enables them to mentor students. If they have done the course, they must have been taught the principles of good mentoring and will be aware

of students' learning needs. Often a mentoring qualification is an expectation when applying for midwifery jobs. So you see that for midwives, working with students is all in a day's (or night's) work and if you are lucky you will be assigned someone who enjoys mentoring. In each placement you attend, you will be allocated a mentor and sometimes you'll be allocated two (see Chapter 3).

Your mentors will be responsible for ensuring you achieve the clinical competencies you have been set by your University and they will be signing these off in your paperwork as you go along. The list of competencies is a useful guide to the skills you are expected to acquire over the academic year. At the start of the year, this list of requirements seems very daunting but if you work at it steadily with your mentors, it should be quite achievable. Perhaps the greatest impact on your development as a student midwife will be the person you work with day to day.

Many mentors are fantastic – they are well informed, up-to-date, keen to teach, open to new ideas, supportive, patient (you will be slow at first), encouraging, wonderful role models and understanding of the pressures on students. A good mentor will be happy to discuss your thoughts and emotions with you and, within the constraints of the work setting, provide an environment where you feel safe to try new things. Because being a midwife is often quite a solitary job, it can be very rewarding as a mentor to share your expertise and insights with someone who is learning. You may, however, come across some of the less appealing types of mentor as (Box 2.1).

Box 2.1 Types of mentors

■ The weary older midwife who is counting down the months to her retirement and has no appetite to pass on what she knows.

■ The mentor who takes advantage of the power the role gives her. She can't be bothered to remember your name and is critical but offers no constructive advice.

■ The fearful hospital midwife who has been subsumed into the NHS hierarchy and tries to draw you into a culture of obedience.

■ The lazy mentor who gets you to do her dirty work.

■ The bossy mentor who takes over and doesn't enable you to learn.

■ The defensive practitioner who is threatened by you and suspicious of any new ideas you may bring from University and so appears dismissive.

As you may imagine, you will have enough demands on you already without having to manage a tricky mentor. You need to take responsibility for your learning needs but it can be difficult to navigate your way around the NHS' complex social structure and develop positive relationships with the staff without a good mentor by your side. It's not just about the mentor, of course. By being positive, amenable, open to learning new things and appreciative of when it's appropriate to ask questions, you are making yourself easy to work with.

If you are experiencing ongoing difficulties working with a mentor, it is important that you speak in confidence to the lecturer at your University who supports students in placements. It is quite possible that you are not the first student to have raised issues about this particular midwife. You may also want to read up on learning styles and maybe try out some quizzes such as Soloman and Felder's 'Index of learning styles questionnaire': http://www.engr.ncsu.edu/learningstyles/ilsweb.html. You and your mentor may be very different people and approach learning in different ways. This can be a useful icebreaker or troubleshooter when it seems the student–mentor relationship may not be working as well as it should.

Multiprofessional/interprofessional working

Your University will probably offer opportunities to learn about multiprofessional teamwork. This may take place in selected modules or possibly in specific sessions when students from a range of health or associated professions share learning together (see Chapters 5 and 7). As soon as you get out into your first placement, the complexities of relationships between health and social care workers from different professions will become apparent. You will come across social workers, neonatal and gynaecological nurses, doctors of all sorts (obstetricians, anaesthetists, cardiologists, endocrinologists, haematologists, GPs etc.), physiotherapists and so on, and you will notice how each group has its own jargon, hierarchy, priorities and entrenched ideas. And all the time you'll be being introduced in practice to the peculiarities of midwifery. If you are already a registered nurse, you will be familiar with multiprofessional/interprofessional working. Use your previous experiences and draw on the skills and expertise you have developed as you get to know the culture of midwifery practice.

The interprofessional learning opportunities invite you to recognise your own discipline's 'tribalism' (Barrett et al. 2005), acknowledge professional differences and then put them aside in order to focus on the needs of the client/patient. While you may hear midwives and social workers say unhelpful things about each other, perhaps the longest standing tensions that exist are between midwives and doctors. Historically, midwifery and obstetrics have grappled over territory and there remain considerable differences between the medical model of birth and midwifery's focus on normality. Medicine has a deep-rooted hierarchical system and some doctors see midwives as obstetric nurses who are there to act on their instruction. This view would put you, in your student midwife's uniform, at the very bottom of the pecking order and this is an uncomfortable place to be.

It is important to remember that, even as a student midwife, you are an advocate for the women in your care

and that midwives don't work *for* doctors but *with* them in an interprofessional team. Put the woman and her baby at the centre of your care, communicate with and access the expertise of other professionals, rise above any pettiness you come across and, if necessary, stand up for yourself and your chosen profession.

Jargon and abbreviations

Midwives and doctors quickly become accustomed to their own peculiar language, and while you will need to pick it up for the sake of effective communication, it will take you some time to be fluent. It would be unreasonable of your mentor to say 'do a BP and a palpation' (translates as take a blood pressure reading and establish how the woman's baby is lying by feeling her abdomen) on your first shift and expect you to understand her. Should you stray into a situation where someone instructs you to 'do an FH' (listen to the fetal heart) or asks for 'a recent Hb' (iron level from a blood sample) or 'an EBL' (estimated blood loss), it is quite acceptable in the early days of your training to ask them to clarify what it is that they would like. In all probability, the woman you are with will be more confused than you are and it is her baby's heart, her iron levels or blood loss that is being discussed.

It will not be long before you are chatting with colleagues about CTGs (cardiotocograph readings of the baby's heart), the EDD (estimated date of delivery) whether calculated by LMP (last menstrual period) or USS (ultrasound scan), SRM (spontaneous rupture of membranes aka someone's waters going), EBM (expressed breast milk), PND (postnatal depression), VBAC (vaginal birth after caesarian) and so on. You will be able to inform your mentor whether the fetus is cephalic (head down) or breech (head up) and if its position is LOA, LOP, LOT, ROA, ROP or ROT. The most important thing is that you can hold on to the memory of your initial bewilderment and let it give you some insight into how disempowering and unsettling the use of incomprehensible jargon and abbreviations is likely to be for the women in your care. You will need to understand obstetric and midwifery language but remember to use it considerately.

Practicalities

Trusts differ in terms of specific uniform requirements for students but while some restrictions are because the hospital Trust wants its staff to look professional, most are because of infection control. Either way, to avoid feeling like a schoolchild told off for your uniform, you may as well observe the rules. If these cause any problems of a religious or cultural nature, then talk to the midwife in charge of the area you are on placement.

Because it can carry infection, jewellery should be kept to a minimum. The rule is usually that you can wear one simple ring (wedding band) without stones, no bracelets, wristwatch, anklets or necklaces and earrings should be small studs or sleepers. Body piercings and tattoos should be discreet and/or covered. Your nails should be clean and cut

reasonably short with no nail varnish. False nails or nail extensions are not permitted (they could fall off and end up somewhere inappropriate or even dangerous). You should wear flat, comfortable shoes which are fully covered (in case someone drops something onto your feet) and well fitting (so you don't fall over). Some Trusts specify that they must be black, although on delivery suite you will probably see quite a range of lurid coloured clogs. You can't wear a cardigan or jumper when doing clinical work, and usually hospital environments are so overheated that you wouldn't want to (avoid wearing a vest for this reason). If your hair is below shoulder length it needs to be tied back and off your collar.

Your identification badge needs to be visible at all times. You may be provided with one by the University or individual Trusts may want you to wear their own. Identification badges will include your photograph and the title 'student midwife'. If you are not used to wearing your name on your clothes, you may initially be surprised that everyone seems to know who you are. Other people's identification badges are invaluable when you are meeting lots of new people, or if you have a bad memory for names, because you can always glance down to see what people are called and what their job is if you are unsure.

The pockets of scrubs, uniform tunics and dresses are surprisingly roomy, so there will be plenty of space for a notebook if you would find one useful. Because documentation is an important part of a midwife's role, you will need a good supply of pens – these must be black as other colours fade over the 25 years maternity notes are stored. It is helpful to have a fob watch pinned to your top so that you can put a time to each documentation entry in the notes and check a woman's pulse or a baby's respirations against the second hand.

Be open-minded and adaptable – eat, drink and use the toilet when you get the chance, even if the timing is not ideal. You don't need to turn into a slave to the machine of hospital midwifery but until you've worked out the structure of the shift and how the next few hours might unfold for you and your mentor, it's best to take opportunities as they arise.

Try to get an understanding of the ward layout and what is kept where early on – this will make you feel more at ease and colleagues will be grateful if you know where to find things (Fig. 2.2).

Support for you in placement

Luisa Cescutti-Butler

If you are concerned about how you will cope whilst in placement, try not to worry as there will be a range of support systems available to you. Your programme handbook will contain a detailed list of the support the University provides. These will not be the same as those that may be available in practice. Read and make a note of the support you think you may need. Ensure that you have all the necessary contact details and don't hesitate to approach the most suitable person if you have any queries or concerns. It is much easier to deal with problems early on than allow them to fester. On occasions, what you see as a problem or issue specific to you may actually have an impact on others (women in your care, fellow students or staff), so it is important that you share these concerns. Fig. 2.3 illustrates what support is available for you whilst you are in practice.

Having a specific learning difference and how this may impact you in the workplace

Dyslexia, dyspraxia and dyscalculia are a number of conditions which are classified under the umbrella term specific learning difference (SpLD) (Cowen 2010); these are classed as a disability under the Equality Act (HMSO 2010). The law requires organisations such as NHS Trust hospitals to promote equality of opportunity and demonstrate positive attitudes towards disability (Cowen 2010). You may not consider yourself as having a disability at all and may have developed strategies to cope with any particular 'weaknesses' you may be affected by; however, there are still reasonable adjustments that organisations are obliged to put in place to help you overcome your difficulties (Cowen 2010). Remember, if you have declared a 'disability', you will still be expected to demonstrate you are 'fit for practice' and meet all the skills and competencies set out in your undergraduate programme (Cowen 2010).

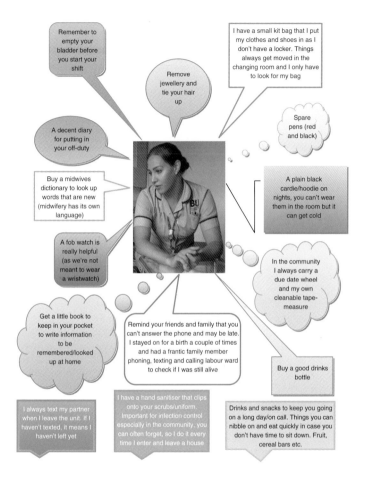

Remember to empty your bladder before you start your shift

Remove jewellery and tie your hair up

I have a small kit bag that I put my clothes and shoes in as I don't have a locker. Things always get moved in the changing room and I only have to look for my bag

Spare pens (red and black)

A decent diary for putting in your off-duty

Buy a midwives dictionary to look up words that are new (midwifery has its own language)

A plain black cardie/hoodie on nights, you can't wear them in the room but it can get cold

A fob watch is really helpful (as we're not meant to wear a wristwatch)

In the community I always carry a due date wheel and my own cleanable tape-measure

Get a little book to keep in your pocket to write information to be remembered/looked up at home

Remind your friends and family that you can't answer the phone and may be late. I stayed on for a birth a couple of times and had a frantic family member phoning, texting and calling labour ward to check if I was still alive

Buy a good drinks bottle

I always text my partner when I leave the unit. If I haven't texted, it means I haven't left yet

I have a hand sanitiser that clips onto your scrubs/uniform. Important for infection control especially in the community, you can often forget, so I do it every time I enter and leave a house

Drinks and snacks to keep you going on a long day/on call. Things you can nibble on and eat quickly in case you don't have time to sit down. Fruit, cereal bars etc.

Figure 2.2 Checklist: preparing for placement.

Very often students find out they have SpLD only once starting at University and after having been through a process of assessment to confirm what it is. The Additional Learning Support team will write to your programme leader advising them on what adjustments need to be made by tutors and

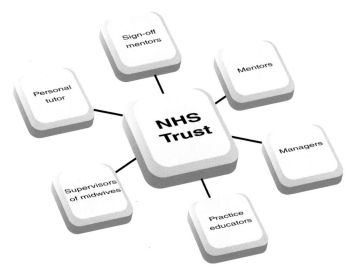

Figure 2.3 Other sources of support.

so on. For example you may get extra time in exams or handouts provided for you before lectures. However, these recommendations are only for the academic environment, there usually are not any suggestions for how you may cope whilst in placement. A pocket guide around dyslexia, dyspraxia and dyscalculia has been produced by the Royal College of Nurses (RCN) and may be a useful resource for you. The guide, which provides an overview of the three conditions specified above including top tips for coping whilst in placement, is easily available through the Internet and may be found at http://www.rcn.org.uk. It also briefly discusses the issue

about whether you should disclose your 'disability'. It is really up to you but it would help if you disclose to your mentors that you have one of the three D's as it will help placement and your mentors to make 'reasonable adjustments'.

Other disabilities

Some students have other forms of disabilities which may be long term and registerable or of a short duration. These may include epilepsy, diabetes, hearing loss or a limb dysfunction (the latter may be temporary due to, for example, a fracture). It is very important that you declare these disabilities as appropriate measures need to be put in place to support you when you are in placement (Disability Discrimination Act 1995) (HMSO 1995). You may need an occupational health referral in order to provide the midwifery staff in the University and clinical area with recommendations for reasonable adjustments such as specific aids, need for regular breaks or restrictions on shifts worked. Your health and well-being are a priority. However, the needs and safety of the women and babies in your care also need to be considered as a priority. You may require a risk assessment and an action plan to be discussed and agreed upon among you, your academic tutor and the clinical manager. At times, some activities which involve greater risk such as use of sharps (needles, amnihooks etc.) or carrying babies may need to be restricted for a period of time until your condition is under control. Please ensure you seek the relevant support if you have any of these conditions or disabilities; we all want to help you to achieve your goal of becoming a midwife within safe and manageable boundaries.

Other sources of support

At times you may find it helpful to seek support from a neutral third party. Your University will provide you with information about counselling and chaplaincy facilities; the Student Union may also be helpful. If all else fails, then you have the option of calling Nightline. It offers 24 hour emotional support for students in distress. If you are having problems that you don't wish to discuss with your personal tutor or your mentors in practice, this may be an option for you. It is manned by students for students. It is entirely confidential and you don't have to provide your name. Further details can be obtained from http://nightline.ac.uk/

Conclusion

Don't be afraid to ask about things you don't understand. Everyone you are working with will have been a student at some point and should be able to empathise. As an adult student, you are responsible for your own learning needs, although do pick your moment as you may get short shrift if you ask about massage techniques in labour during an obstetric emergency. There is a lot to take in when you first come across any midwifery environment so don't expect to understand everything immediately. Give yourself time to observe what is going on around you, absorb new information and ways of seeing and doing things and get a sense of what is expected of you (Box 2.2). If you have any additional needs/specific learning differences or a disability that may impact you in placement, please don't be afraid of sharing it with your mentor so that reasonable adjustments can be made to help support you in the best possible way. Most importantly, don't lose your sense of why you came into midwifery in the first place, your core beliefs and your concern for the women and babies in your care (see Vignette 2.1). Be yourself, hold onto your ideals and don't let the system swallow you up.

Box 2.2 Top tips from students @ Bournemouth University

First years:

■ Ensure you do read around subject areas

■ Ensure when you are on placement you get involved where you can as the second year comes round far too quickly

■ Ask questions, it's amazing how much information and knowledge you can gain by asking questions

■ Keep your head down and take it all in before you make any decisions about anything!

■ Make the most of every opportunity that comes along, be keen and don't forget to write down everything you do and get your *pad* filled in as soon as possible after the event

■ Don't be intimidated by midwives no matter how they come across, and make friends with MCAs as they know *loads* and can always find things!

■ Enjoy yourselves and share your experiences – keep talking to your peers and your partners – don't remove yourself just because you're not at unit for a while – you are the best support network for each other!

■ If given the opportunity to do something, do it. Having a go at things with supervision enables you to practice skills.

■ My top tip for community/anywhere is to have an alphabetical notebook (like an address book) and write all the handy things in that you might forget (an appt gestations) and so on.

■ Anything new you learn that day – go home and read over it that evening, it consolidates and links your theory to practice and stays in your mind more

■ Don't be afraid to ask midwives questions and research more in depth when you get home. Communication is the key, listen to your colleagues, meet other professionals and be yourself. Also talk to your fellow students in first year and above to share info to learn from each other

Second years:

■ Be proactive

■ You will get down; you may even cry but keep calm and carry on

- Start learning your pregnancy conditions and do a few calculations a week

- Don't give up

- Even if you fail a unit, seek help and look to your peers for support. If they are good friends, they will support and help you

- Do all academic work as it is handed out, and bite the bullet, do the things in practice that you feel uncomfortable about

- Have regular tutorials/contact with tutors and mentors

- Manage your time well, plan out what you intend to do

- Talk to your mentor at the beginning of each shift about what you need more experience in/need to achieve

- Be mega organised!!

- Challenge your weaknesses

- Don't leave everything until the last minute – a little bit often

- Be ambitious

- Don't lose focus or drive, Trust that all the hard work will pay off (it does)

- Don't leave anything until the last minute

- Stay calm and take time out to relax and socialise

- Be confident – you can do it

- Enjoy, you can do it. Good luck

Third years:

- Third year goes very quickly

- Push yourself to work outside of your comfort zone

- Don't panic about getting your 40 births – you will get them

- Use your tutors when applying for jobs

- Even when times are tough, enjoy as much as you can as time will fly!

- Ensure you work over your hours to cater for the unexpected, i.e. sickness or family occasions. And remember to enjoy it and drink lots of wine!

Vignette 2.1 It's only a room?

There's a room in the corridor that's full of fear; a cold tiled shell of technology.

Steely instruments are lined up; soldiers of war; counted and correct; numbered in rank.

The room is considered unnatural, medical and frightening by all.

It's a place full of blood and where scars are created,

Physical and emotional, but permanent all the same.

She considers how her body has let her down.

"What did I do wrong?" is her mantra, as she shivers uncontrollably.

"Something's amiss and our family is threatened".

Comforts are very few, as a wave of failure throws her about like a tiny dinghy in a stormy sea.

She feels unable to protect the most important person in her world.

Trolleys that cannot be touched wheel into view; like crocodiles circling their prey.

Strangers, whose titles she cannot pronounce, do not make eye contact;

But speak an unknown language to each other.

She has little idea what they will do or why.

Hope is now fading very fast as another deep pain takes over from the physical.

The spotlight pierces down, reflecting on the table, bouncing sharply around the room.

The mattress feels hard and she is a vision of torture.

Uncaring exposure elicits vulnerability, as a sheet blinds her from what is happening,

Creating a final curtain as muffled masked voices make no sense.

Sterile liquid drips slowly and her head feels full and frozen.

As her midwife smiles down, she can feel empathy and see the kindness.

Her presence says silently that this is a place where her family will be safe.

The connection is a calming one, that will stay and support.

She feels radiating comfort, courage and caring wash over her.

Someone to share, understand and be there no matter what challenge lays ahead.

The unpronounceable people are now experts,

Their eyes focused only on protecting her and her child.

Muffled voices soothe as they communicate and plan so well with each other.

The table feels warm and comfortable as the spotlight beams down,

Softly highlighting the most important appearance of a very special person; the starring role.

Realisation dawns that she did nothing wrong . . .

Nature needed a helping hand and companions to share the burden.

Determination wells up as a cry rings out and her body feels amazing and strong.

It's a wonderful achievement to create and grow such a life,

And the scars will fade into evidence of motherhood and love.

A slippery pink wriggling bundle is placed on her chest; warm and beautifully heavy.

As the room bursts into comfortable excited chattering,

The midwife smiles down again and their eyes meet.

A moment of joy and pride is shared between mother and midwife.

Both know that they are honoured and grateful to be together at that very moment.

There is a room in the corridor that is full of joy, miracles and challenges.

It is shiny and brightly wrapped in birthday paper, with a very special gift inside.

A warm womb full of caring, compassion, competence, communication and commitment;

Where courage is needed, but can be shared and supported

As this wonderful new life and new hopes for the future begin.

Alison Peters
First-year student, Bournemouth University, Dorset, UK
Reproduced with permission of Alison Peters

References

Barkley A (2011) Ideals, expectations and reality: challenges for student midwives. *Br J Midwifery* 19: 259–264.

Barrett G, Sellman D, Thomas J (2005) *Interprofessional Working in Health and Social Care: Professional Perspectives*. Palgrave Macmillan, Basingstoke.

Bosanquet A (2002) "Stones can make people docile": reflections of a student midwife on how the hospital environment makes "good girls". *MIDIRS Midwifery Digest* 12: 301–305.

Cowen M. (2010) Dyslexia, dyspraxia + dyscalculia: a tool kit for nursing staff. Available at http://www.rcn.org.uk (last accessed 21 August 2014).

HMSO (1995) The Disability Discrimination Act. Available at http://www.nidirect.gov.uk/the-disability-discrimination-act-dda (last accessed 1 September 2014).

HMSO (2010) *Her Majesty's Stationery Office (2010) Equality Act*. HMSO, London.

Health and Safety Executive (2006) *Managing Shift Work: Health and Safety Guidance*. HSE, Bootle.

Lee K, Busby A (2010) Going to University: hints and tips for new midwifery students. *Br J Midwifery* 18: 66–67.

Further resources

The British Dyslexia Association: http://www.bda-dyslexia.org.uk.

Dyslexia Action: http://www.dyslexia-inst.org.uk.

The Dyspraxia Foundation: http://www.dyspraxiafoundation.org.uk.

The Dyscalculia Centre: http://www.dyscalculia.me.uk.

Chapter 3
ASSESSMENT OF PRACTICE

Margaret Fisher

Introduction

The Nursing and Midwifery Council (NMC 2009) requires practice to be assessed in all pre-registration midwifery programmes. A minimum of 50% of your programme will be spent in practice and its assessment is therefore a hugely important aspect of your preparation to become a midwife. Not only is practice an essential part of the preparation of midwives from a professional body perspective, but recognition for its contribution to overall degree classification is gaining importance. Valuing practice in this way therefore benefits you as a student (rewarding excellence), recognises those supporting you in practice and raises the profile of the profession. Increasingly women and their partners or families are being asked to contribute to the assessment of practice, and programme teams have developed a range of methods of capturing this vital perspective.

The Nursing and Midwifery Council 'Standards to support learning and assessment in practice' (NMC 2008a) and 'Standards for pre-registration midwifery education' (NMC 2009) are the main professional documents which set the requirements for practice assessment. Both are currently being reviewed so there may be changes to these in the future – it is important you keep up-to-date with any new publications. This chapter explains the standards, principles, terminology and processes. It is divided into sections which include the following:

- Purpose

- Process

- Positives

- Pitfalls

- Preparation

As can be seen in my biography, practice assessment and mentorship are of particular personal interest. Findings from several projects in which I have been involved have been included in this chapter where appropriate.

The Hands-on Guide to Midwifery Placements, First Edition.
Edited by Luisa Cescutti-Butler and Margaret Fisher.
© 2016 John Wiley & Sons, Ltd. Published 2016 by John Wiley & Sons, Ltd.

These comprise my Masters dissertation on midwifery mentors (Fisher & Webb 2008; Fisher 2009); a 5-year study of practice assessment in midwifery, social work and emergency care programmes referred to as 'CEPPL' – the Centre for Excellence in Professional Placement Learning – a government-funded Centre at Plymouth University (CEPPL 2011; Fisher et al. 2011); and a recent scoping activity of practice assessment processes in midwifery programmes throughout the United Kingdom (Bower et al. 2014; Fisher et al. 2015). References and electronic links to publications can be found at the end of the chapter for further reading.

This chapter will also explain the Fitness to Practise procedure which may, on occasions, be invoked if concerns are raised about a student's conduct or health when on a midwifery or nursing programme. The relevance of this to practice assessment will be discussed, along with links to other chapters in the book.

You may find the information a bit much to start with – so perhaps dip in and out until you are clear on the roles and processes and have some practice experience on which to pin it.

Purpose

Why does practice need to be *assessed*? It is important that you understand the reason for this; otherwise it runs the risk of being seen simply as a 'tick-box exercise' which adds to workload without any clear purpose (Fisher et al. 2011). The NMC's requirement for midwifery practice to be awarded a grade which contributes to academic credits and therefore degree classification may be seen as a tangible outcome for students. This has gone some way to raising the profile of practice, and acknowledging its value (Bower et al. 2014; Fisher et al. 2015). It has, however, also made students very competitive and resulted in some losing sight of the true purpose. It is important to move beyond the numerical value and look at what is *really* being assessed and what this means. The assessment document will include a set of criteria, based on NMC requirements including skills, knowledge and attributes which you must achieve in order to progress to the next stage of your programme or be deemed fit to go on the register (more of this later). How well you are performing in relation to these criteria is vital for you to know so that you can work on any areas which are weaker while maintaining and continuing to improve those aspects in which you are stronger. The whole purpose is to ensure that you are practising in a way which is leading towards you becoming a safe, competent and confident midwife. Importantly, you need to realise that it is your *performance* which is being assessed and not you as an individual. Your *personality* will of course influence your performance, but you yourself are not being judged.

You may have your own views as to how well you are doing, but it is important to get feedback from practitioners who know what this professional registration really means. Of course, your sign-off mentors are all individuals and some are more effective at this role than others. Chapter 2 has highlighted how mentors can vary, although you will find that the vast majority are excellent and take the role very seriously (Fisher & Webb 2008; Fisher 2009). It is therefore important that the assessment tool used is fit for purpose and supports those measuring your performance to do so in as consistent and objective way as possible (Fisher et al. 2011). Midwifery programme teams around the country are currently trying to learn 'best practice' from each other, establishing a set of key principles and potentially a common grading matrix which can be modified to meet individual institutional requirements and curricula to further enhance this process (Lead Midwife for Education-UK group; Bower et al. 2014; Fisher et al. 2015). Some of the 'processes' discussed in the next section seek to overcome these variations, but because the complexity of humanity is involved there is inevitably going to be an element of subjectivity in your assessment.

This is where you need to focus on the *purpose*. Although you may want to have a grade in the 90's but your sign-off mentor thinks you should receive 70%, the overall message is that you are achieving, and doing so at a very high level. This should be of greatest importance to you in that your assessment is telling you that you are well on the way to becoming an excellent midwife. Likewise, if you are receiving a grade which is barely a pass, the clear message is that you need to do a lot of work in order to succeed in practice. You need to be

discussing some key learning objectives with your sign-off mentor and personal tutor to ensure you are going to ultimately meet the requirements for registration as a midwife.

It is also very important for you to develop self-awareness, and the practice assessment process can encourage this. Sophie Denning, a second year midwifery student at Plymouth University (PU), says that it is important that you

'Understand your role as a student midwife and what mentors will expect from you.'

Even if your programme does not require formal self-assessment, make sure that you regularly review your progress against the set criteria and *honestly* measure your performance. If you have any doubts that you are 'making the grade' then speak to your sign-off mentor or personal tutor urgently and ask them to help you to devise an action plan to address any weaknesses. You might like to try out the hypothetical activity in Box 3.1. It is much easier for you to do this if you have personally acknowledged that you have difficulties than if someone has told you so; the motivation to improve will be much stronger (think of the principle of Alcoholics Anonymous). Self-awareness is a hugely important attribute to develop and will make you a much safer and better professional. 'Making Practice-Based Learning Work' (Marsh et al. 2015) is a useful resource designed for those supporting learning in practice, but also with some handy hints if there are any issues about your achievement in practice (though I am sure you won't need this).

> **Box 3.1** Action plan scenario
>
> You are three weeks into your first placement in community. Julie, your sign-off mentor, meets with you to discuss your progress. She says that you seem to be struggling in antenatal clinics. You don't appear to find it easy to relate to the women and are very hesitant in performing abdominal palpations.
>
> Think about
>
> ■ What verbal and non-verbal 'messages' may you be demonstrating to give this impression?
>
> ■ Why may you be behaving in this way?
>
> ■ What actions do you need to take to make progress in this area in the remaining three weeks of your placement?

Process

The NMC provides the *principles* for practice assessment but individual midwifery programmes will differ in their translation of these into specific documents and processes. There will, however, be elements which are common to all and will be explained further in this section:

a. Practice placements

b. Sign-off mentor (and perhaps co/buddy/associate mentors)

c. Ongoing Achievement Record

d. Assessment document

e. Grading of practice

f. Practice progress review meetings (usually referred to as 'tripartites' or 'triads')

Practice placements

These are of course fundamental to your programme, enabling you to learn, practise and refine the various clinical skills and professional behaviours which will be needed as a midwife. The fact that this book has been written is testament to the importance of practice placements in your midwifery course. It is, however, important that you recognise that the placements actually exist for the purpose of service to the public. You will be supported in experiencing a range of learning opportunities, but the needs of the service may at times conflict with your plans, and the former will take priority.

Other chapters in this book such as those covering 'Low risk', 'High risk' and 'Wider experiences' highlight the various placements and models of care you are likely to encounter as a midwifery student. Read these carefully to see how you can best plan your placement around the requirements of your practice assessments; devise appropriate learning objectives which will make best use of any specific learning opportunities and use your practice assessment document to focus on particular outcomes relevant to that placement. Discuss these with your sign-off mentor.

Audit and evaluation

The NMC requires all clinical areas in which midwifery (or nursing) students are placed to be audited as suitable learning environments (NMC 2008a). This is a partnership activity undertaken regularly by clinicians and academics. Part of this process will require student evaluations of placements to be completed. It is very important that you do this in an honest and detailed fashion, including both positive and constructive criticism. Please make sure that you let your personal tutor or an appropriate clinical staff member (ward or department manager or someone with responsibility for education) know if there is anything which needs attention. Take ownership of your feedback; it is part of becoming an accountable practitioner (see also the sections on escalating concerns in Chapters 1 and 5). Students are not able to be placed (and therefore assessed) in areas which are not appropriate and where there are insufficient or inadequately prepared sign-off mentors.

Sign-off mentor

This will be a *very* important person to you in every placement. It is the sign-off mentor who will be monitoring and assessing your progress while also (usually) being your main 'teacher' and 'advisor' and co-ordinating your learning activities. The role of 'sign-off mentor' was introduced by the NMC in 2006 and became a mandatory requirement in 2008 ('Standards to support learning and assessment in practice', NMC 2008a). This built on and formalised the previous role of the 'mentor' who was required to:

> ' . . . facilitate learning and supervise[s] and
> assess[es] students in the practice setting'
> English National Board for Nursing,
> Midwifery and Health Visiting
> (2001, p6)

A number of factors gave rise to this more formal role including an unacceptably high number of recently qualified nurses and midwives falling foul of the NMC Code of conduct and needing to be investigated at Fitness to Practise hearings (see the section at the end of this chapter for further explanation). They commissioned a study into why mentors 'fail to fail' students (Duffy 2004), and this concept has continued to be discussed in more recent literature (Rutkowski 2007; Jervis & Tilki 2011). As a result, the NMC increased the emphasis on the accountability of the role. Along with this, the requirements for those responsible for assessing nursing and midwifery students as fit to go on the register were tightened up. Look at Box 3.2 which lists these requirements. Because of the nature of midwifery and its statutory role as well as the degree of autonomy qualified midwives have, it was considered that a 'sign-off mentor' was in fact required throughout the programme, at all 'progression points' (NMC 2009). This differs from nursing in which a sign-off mentor is currently only required in the student's final placement, although it is possible that this may align with midwifery in the future.

Box 3.2   Requirements of sign-off mentors

Nurses and midwives who intend to take on the role of *mentor* must fulfil the following criteria:

■ Be registered in the same part or sub-part of the register as the student they are to assess and for the nurses' part of the register to be in the same field of practice.

■ Have developed their own knowledge, skills and competence beyond registration, that is, been registered for at least 1 year.

■ Have successfully completed an NMC approved mentor preparation programme.

■ Have the ability to select, support and assess a range of learning opportunities in their area of practice for students undertaking NMC approved programmes.

■ Be able to support learning in an interprofessional environment – selecting and supporting a range of learning opportunities for students from other professions.

■ Have the ability to contribute to the assessment of other professionals under the supervision of an experienced assessor from that profession.

■ Be able to make judgements about competence/proficiency of NMC students on the same part of the register, and in the same field of practice, and be accountable for such decisions.

■ Be able to support other nurses and midwives in meeting CPD needs in accordance with the Code: Standards for conduct, performance and ethics for nurses and midwives.

A nurse or midwife designated to *sign-off* proficiency for a particular student at the end of a programme must additionally have

■ Clinical currency and capability in the field in which the student is being assessed

■ A working knowledge of current programme requirements, practice assessment strategies and relevant changes in education and practice for the student they are assessing

■ An understanding of the NMC registration requirements and the contribution they make to the achievement of these requirements

(continued)

What this means to you is that you will find that you have midwifery sign-off mentors allocated to you for the majority of your course, and it will be essential that they are the people who assess whether or not you have achieved at each progression point or on completion of the programme (NMC 2008a, 2009). You are expected to work 'under direct or indirect supervision' of your sign-off mentor for at least 40% of your practice time (equating to usually 2 days per week minimum). Note that your sign-off mentor can liaise with others who have worked with you; they do not have to physically work with you on every shift. This allows for periods of annual leave or part-time staff, for example. If they have an additional role (such as a manager) which means that they cannot work directly with you as much, it is their responsibility to ensure they talk to your co-mentors so that they can assess your progress.

Likewise, as you advance through your programme you will undertake more practice under reducing levels of supervision. An analogy I use when teaching Mentorship is the elastic lead used for dogs (Fig. 3.1). To start with, you need to be working immediately alongside your sign-off mentor (or supervising midwife). Gradually, you will move away from them and undertake periods of care with them indirectly supervising you. On some occasions you may even be working out of sight (e.g., when doing your caseloading – see Chapter 6). You are, however, always 'attached' to your sign-off mentor and you can come swiftly back to them or they can follow you if, for example, a low-risk situation becomes high risk. The 'elastic lead' of their registration number and therefore accountability for your practice – actions and omissions – will not be released until you complete your programme and are practising under your own PIN (Personal Identification Number). It is therefore a hugely responsible role to be a sign-off mentor, and you need to appreciate that different midwives will be happier to let that lead stretch than others; much will be

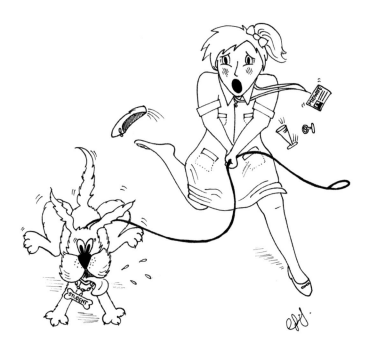

Figure 3.1 Analogy for appropriate level of supervision by mentors. Reproduced with permission of Clare Shirley, third-year midwifery student, Bournemouth University.

down to their confidence in you, so it is important that you let them watch you until they are reassured of your capabilities, and make sure you always keep them informed about what you are thinking and actions you are proposing. If you are already registered as a nurse, it is extremely important to remember that you are practising under your midwifery mentor's registration and not your own as a nurse during your pre-registration midwifery programme. You must therefore follow the same principles.

Buddy/associate/co-mentors

In many placements, you may also have one or more designated buddy/associate/co-mentors allocated to you (terminology will vary in different areas). It can be very valuable to have nominated additional midwives helping to support your learning and providing you with wider experiences and role modeling. The team approach can also provide you with more continuity of mentorship, e.g., when your sign-off mentor is on annual leave. It is likely that your co-mentors will also be invited to contribute to the evidence supporting the decision of the sign-off mentor as to whether or not you have achieved in practice. In many instances, your co-mentor may be working towards becoming a sign-off mentor themselves, so it is important you work with them and try to invite them to your tripartite/practice review meetings if your programme allows for this. You may also find you receive a higher grade due to their verbal and written contributions adding to the pool of evidence.

Ongoing achievement record (OAR)

The NMC requires all midwifery students to have some form of practice record which is transferred between separate placements or clinical allocations (see NMC 2009 p22). This enables all those involved in your assessment to be able to see how you have progressed and contributes to the evidence for subsequent placements. In most cases, this will take the format of a practice portfolio which may be paper-based, electronic or a blended mixture. It may include the following:

- Learning objectives

- Reflections

- Comments from others

- Evidence of wider reading or attendance at extra-curricula study sessions

- Record of European Union (EU) numbers (NMC 2009)

- Your assessment document

It will be a document which you will guard with your life.

Box 3.3 shows Keri's 'Top Tips' for maintaining your OAR:

Box 3.3   Top tips for your portfolio of evidence

- "Look at the learning criteria for each section of the portfolio when writing your learning objectives for the placement. It will help you to achieve the outcomes and provides your mentor with a structure for your learning.

- Make sure you get experiences signed off in your practice portfolio by the member of staff you have worked with on the day, and update your online portfolio as soon after the event as possible."

Keri Morter
Second-year student, Plymouth University, Plymouth, UK
Reproduced with permission of Keri Morter.

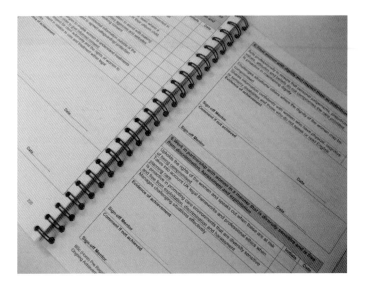

Figure 3.2 Example of a practice assessment document.

Assessment document

This may form part of your OAR or be a separate document (Fig. 3.2). The NMC has set out key elements which must be explicitly assessed in both theory and practice. The 'Standards for pre-registration midwifery education' (NMC 2009) explain the Midwifery Competencies and Essential Skills Clusters in detail (see also Chapter 1), but in summary they comprise the following:

Competencies (Standard 17, categorized as 'Domains' on pages 23–35)

■ Effective midwifery practice

■ Professional and ethical practice

■ Developing the individual midwife and others

■ Achieving quality care through evaluation and research.

Essential skills clusters (see pages 35–67)

■ Communication

■ Initial consultation between the woman and the midwife

■ Normal labour and birth

■ Initiation and continuance of breastfeeding

■ Medicines management

Future revision of the Standards may see some changes in terminology/ content – but it is likely that these elements will remain core to practice assessment.

You will find that your midwifery programme assessment document will map the skills, attributes and knowledge which are being assessed to these elements. The method of doing this will vary (Bower et al. 2014; Fisher et al. 2015). In most cases, assessment will be 'continuous' – in other words your sign-off mentor will be monitoring your progress throughout your daily practice against set criteria. This will either be through working with you themselves or communicating with others who have been supervising you. Some programmes may include focused assessments of specific skills or activities, and you will be advised if this is the case and how best to prepare for them. There will be 'progression points' when completion of all relevant criteria will be measured and your development during that stage of the programme will be assessed. All midwifery students will therefore have demonstrated achievement of these professional requirements in order to be assessed as competent and fit for entry to the register on completion of the programme. Georgia Moffatt, second-year student at Plymouth University says that:

> 'Discussing with [my] mentor about how things are going constantly helps me understand where I am, and where I am going in regards to my learning objectives.'

As you can imagine, documentation of your development and achievement will take time. It is vitally important to keep up with this, otherwise it becomes a struggle for both you and your sign-off mentor and the purpose also becomes eroded. If you leave all your paperwork until the time of your assessment, you will indeed feel that it is a 'tick-box exercise' and heavy workload. You may also find that the quality of both the evidence and the assessment itself is not as good. Busy practice and academic staff will become frustrated and irritated if documentation is not completed at the required time, and resultant delays in your assessment meeting will have a knock-on effect to other appointments and commitments.

Protected time

Acknowledging the associated workload and the importance of value being given to the assessment process and appropriate judgements being made, the NMC set out in their Standards (NMC 2009) the requirement for an hour per week of 'protected time' with your sign-off mentor to review your progress. This was designed to enable you to discuss your working towards your objectives for that placement, undertake focused learning and keep the relevant documentation up-to-date. In reality, you will find that it is near-impossible to achieve this on a weekly basis. When you are in a community setting you will generally find that you have more time (car journeys are very useful) to discuss how you are doing as you go along, however when you are placed in a busy maternity unit it can be extremely difficult to get together on a regular basis due to service commitments and shift patterns. What you and your sign-off mentor need to acknowledge is that protected time will not just 'happen'. It will take planning and organisation in order to achieve it. You will also need the support of the rest of the team – and they should be prepared to do this as part of their communal responsibility towards education in practice (Fisher & Webb 2008). Although the needs of the women and service must always take priority, with sufficient structured planning you should be able to achieve this on a reasonably regular basis. Discuss with your sign-off mentor:

■ What is the unit/Trust approach to meeting this NMC requirement? Do they explicitly acknowledge the importance of it and are there any existing arrangements to help sign-off mentors and students to meet? Do they make allowances for sign-off mentors to have this time available during working hours or do they offer 'time in lieu' or a financial alternative if it is not possible to achieve this in usual hours?

■ Is there an expectation as to how this should be documented?

■ Is an hour a week appropriate or would a more flexible approach be easier, e.g., such as: half an hour twice a week or a couple of hours a fortnight?

■ What time of day tends to be better? Is there a period when there is overlap of shifts and therefore more staff on duty, or the area tends to be a little quieter?

■ What are your sign-off mentor's personal commitments (work and home life)?

■ Look at the off-duty and check any 'booked' activities (if relevant to the clinical area) and staffing levels; identify suitable dates and times and write them on the off-duty next to both of your names (check you are allowed to do this with the local rostering system).

■ Discuss where to meet – it is usually best to take yourselves away from your usual work environment so that you are less likely to be disturbed. This is where the team's support comes in – they need to know when and where you are both going and may be able to cover more urgent work in your absence.

■ Make sure you have all of your documentation ready for the meeting; this will make best use of the time and show your sign-off mentor that you are proactive about your learning. They and the team will be more supportive towards you if they know that you are making good use of these periods.

Remember that your sign-off mentor will have a range of other responsibilities in addition to mentoring you. Please treat them with consideration and respect and approach requests with diplomacy. Help them to fulfil their role by ensuring you communicate clearly, are proactive about arranging any meetings and provide them with documentation at their request so that they are able to keep this up to date.

Grading of practice

The NMC requires practice to be awarded a grade which contributes to the credits leading to the academic award (Standard 15 – Assessment Strategy, NMC 2009, p 20–21). In some programmes this will be a specific mark or percentage; in others a classification such as AA, A, BB, B and C may be used. A matrix or guide for grading against specific criteria is likely to be included in your practice assessment documentation. In most programmes, the sign-off mentor will be responsible for awarding the practice grade – although this may vary between institutions as some combine or replace this with input from academic staff; the sign-off mentor comments or individual assessment tasks providing the evidence needed to determine the ultimate grade awarded (Fisher et al. 2015).

The level at which you are expected to perform will increase each year – and you may find your practice grades therefore decrease if you do not work at a higher level, for instance dealing with more complexity or taking more of a lead in referring any deviations from normal. This reflects what happens in your academic assessments. In some institutions practice-related activities such as reflections may also contribute to the practice grade (Bower et al. 2014; Fisher et al. 2015).

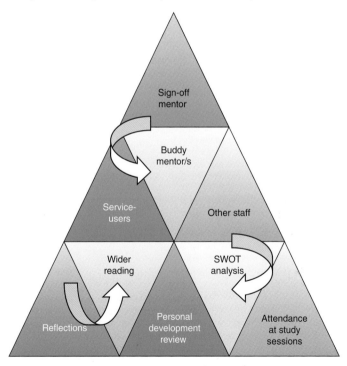

Figure 3.3 Triangulation of practice assessment.

Triangulation of evidence

The NMC (2009) requires the grade awarded to be based on clear evidence, and you will find that the process of documenting this will again vary in format in different programmes. Popular sources of evidence include reflections, learning from in-house or external study days and wider reading. You are also strongly encouraged to gain as many written accounts as you can from a range of other individuals with whom you have worked (whether midwives or other professionals or support workers) as well as the women or families for whom you have cared. This 'triangulation of evidence' has been shown to be very beneficial in gaining a more accurate reflection of abilities and performance, enhancing the reliability of assessment (Fig. 3.3) (Fisher et al. 2011). It is also a very important aspect of a registrant's practice, and has been included in the new 'The Code' (NMC 2015, standard 9.2) as part of the revalidation process. You may also find your grades are higher if you are able to provide a number of positive accounts from others. Please seek guidance from your programme team as to how best to access and document this evidence. Self-assessment and personal development techniques such as SWOT analysis (Strengths, Weaknesses, Opportunities, Threats), learning objectives and capability or professional development plans will also form a valuable contribution to this pool of evidence – see some useful websites at the end of this chapter. Think broadly. Victoria Shaw, first-year student at Plymouth University, shares the value of taking this proactive approach to her practice learning in Vignette 3.1.

Vignette 3.1 Identifying your learning needs

"When first going out into placement each student is expected to undertake a SWOT analysis. The aim of this is to detect our own strengths, weaknesses, opportunities and threats. I decided that one of my weaknesses was my lack of clinical experience; I was worried that by not having any past experience it may put me behind others when it came to going out on placement. Although it is massively exciting to be going out on placement only 10 weeks into the course, it's extremely nerve-racking. I know in previous years the students didn't go out into practice until February, which means they had those extra weeks to practise their clinical skills before going on placement. Having been on placement for only a week I feel more confident in these already. It is evident to me that clinical skills can only really be taught and learnt thoroughly in the workplace. Practising them before going out on placement was helpful, in the sense that I had a rough idea of how to carry out some clinical tasks. In actual fact, it was through practising in the real environment of the hospital that I really cemented my knowledge and had the opportunity to master some of these skills. I feel that learning practical skills whilst out on placement makes it a lot more real and I now have an

(continued)

understanding and appreciation of why they are done and how important they are. For example, learning how to do a set of observations; each time they are done they form the basis of a bigger picture.

The best advice I can give any new students preparing to go out on their first placement is to decide what your own strengths and weaknesses are. Make sure you have a clear idea in your mind of what it is you need to work on when you go onto placement, this way when a midwife asks you what it is you are hoping to learn from your first placement you have an answer for them. This will enable you to get the most out of your placement and have a clear idea of your learning objectives from the outset."

Victoria Shaw
First-year student, Plymouth University
Reproduced with permission of Victoria Shaw.

Practice progress review meetings (tripartites/triads)

It is highly likely that you will find that review meetings form part of the practice assessment process in your institution. In most Universities, this is called a 'tripartite' or 'triad' (Bower et al. 2014; Fisher et al. 2015). These normally take the form of a three-way discussion about your progress in practice between your sign-off mentor, an academic midwife such as your personal tutor and yourself, but a wide range of variations exist throughout the United Kingdom (Fisher et al. 2015). Conversations may take place over the telephone or via e-mail. The majority of institutions, however, prefer face-to-face discussions as this is probably the most rigorous of the approaches. Disadvantages are that they can be problematic to arrange and are resource-intensive (Fisher et al. 2011). As a result, some programmes choose to rely on written evidence from sign-off mentors and an academic tutor

will meet with the student to review their documentation and perhaps combine this with awarding a grade (Fisher et al. 2015). You may also be required to contribute to your own assessment.

The timings of these tripartite or practice progress meetings will vary, and some or all of the following may be used in your institution (Bower et al. 2014; Fisher et al. 2015):

■ at the beginning of a placement to discuss learning objectives and any issues;

■ midpoint to discuss progress to date and how well you are moving towards achieving the objectives/criteria;

■ at the end of a placement or at a specific time in the year when 'summative' assessment (i.e., determination of achievement or grading) takes place.

The role of the academic in these meetings is generally accepted as

■ ensuring you and your sign-off mentor understand the documentation;

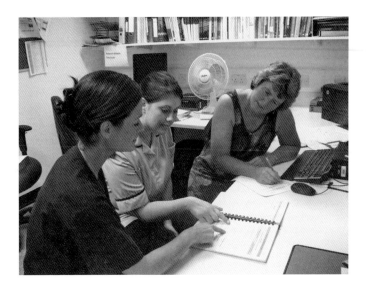

Figure 3.4 Tripartite meeting.

■ monitoring your progress towards the defined criteria for the stage in your programme;

■ ensuring that the evidence is available in your documentation;

■ ensuring that any grades awarded reflect the evidence available – that is, moderate any awarded by the sign-off mentor or ensure that commentary reflects that required by the programme so that the academic can award the appropriate grade;

■ providing support to the sign-off mentor in making their decisions.

Organising these meetings (Fig. 3.4) is a very important part of your practice assessment process. If your programme

allows it, and the other attendees are happy, please remember to invite your co-mentors.

Although the description above is the usual interpretation of a tripartite meeting, some programmes may use this term in an alternative way (Bower et al. 2014; Fisher et al. 2015). The people present most often include you, your personal tutor or academic assessor and a clinician (usually your sign-off mentor). However, the purpose may not be a review of your progress but instead a specific practice assessment. Read Lou Ellis' account of setting up her practice assessment 'tripartite' at Bournemouth University in *Vignette 3.2*, and the learning she has gained about the value of self-assessment and assertiveness in this process:

Vignette 3.2 A practice assessment

'My first assessment by a mentor was my postnatal tripartite which is an assessment on a postnatal examination of both mother and baby. This was conducted in the middle of my first year of training. To make the assessment easier for myself, I chose a mother and baby who were low risk and who had both required minimal care and support. The woman had had her baby 7 days ago and was nearing the time for discharge from midwifery care. I was extremely nervous, in fact petrified of messing up as not only was my mentor to be present but also my academic advisor. I didn't get much sleep the days leading up to the assessment.

The day of the assessment arrived. We had received a message stating that on day 5 the woman's blood pressure was raised and she was feeling unwell and didn't know if she would be up to an assessment. This left me panicked as I did not want to do an assessment on a woman I hadn't previously met as I wasn't confident, and the idea of rearranging was devastating as it had taken weeks to pin down both my academic advisor and my mentor. However, after speaking with the woman she was feeling much better and as her blood pressure was normal the day before she was happy for the visit to go ahead.

Although I was glad the assessment was going ahead I was now nervous as my nice low-risk assessment could potentially be more complicated. I remember shaking as I was walking to the house. Both my mentor and academic advisor were reassuring and supportive which helped. The visit was going well, I had checked the woman over and had just started checking her baby when I realised I hadn't washed my hands in between her and her baby. I verbalised this and got up and washed my hands. The visit went well with no other concerns. The assessment then needed to be marked between myself, my mentor and my academic advisor. I found it very difficult to mark myself as I knew that I had made a mistake by not washing my hands in between the mother and baby examination, and at that moment in time I was unable to see past my mistake and look at the areas that I had excelled in. In the end I just agreed with the overall mark that my mentor and academic advisor came up with as I lacked the confidence to discuss my good points.

Over the course of the 3 years I have had the opportunities to assess my own and others' work through similar assessments and I am now able to discuss which areas I have excelled in and which areas I feel that I need to improve in. This experience has been invaluable to me throughout my training as I am now able to reflect back on everyday situations and learn from them. Conducting tripartite assessments has given me the confidence to openly discuss with mentors and even challenge them if I feel I am being marked unfairly, especially if they don't look at the marking criteria first. What I learnt from this experience is that we are only human and everyone makes mistakes. This is okay as long as we recognise and learn from it. I've also learnt that it is important to recognise when you have done well and to be proud when you receive a high mark as it is often well deserved. The last 3 years have been a real learning curve for me, and now that I am nearly qualified I know that the real learning begins.'

Lou Ellis
Third-year student, Bournemouth University, Poole, UK
Reproduced with permission of Lou Ellis.

Positives

Practice assessment provides you with many positive outcomes which include:

■ A structure to your programme, helping you to build on your knowledge and experience

■ An opportunity to see how far you have come and to celebrate achievements

■ Praise and encouragement

■ Increased confidence in your abilities

■ Value given to your efforts and all those sacrifices you have had to make

■ Reassurance that you are making progress towards or achieving the required criteria to become a registered midwife

■ Can improve your overall profile towards your degree classification.

The CEPPL study on Assessment of Practice (Fisher et al. 2011) specifically looked at Plymouth University midwifery students' experiences of *tripartites* (progress meetings) as one of the assessment methods, and students commented that they:

■ Helped to clarify and focus learning objectives and expectations

■ Were useful checkpoints

■ Helped them to reflect

■ Provided an opportunity to clarify issues

■ Enabled constructive feedback to be given

■ Provided a useful forum for discussion with their sign-off mentor and personal tutor

■ Provided an opportunity to raise any concerns

■ Were generally found to be supportive, relaxed and friendly.

Observed assessments similar to the one described by Lou in *Vignette 3.2* were experienced by social work students in this study. They were found to have the following advantages:

■ Students benefiting from the opportunity to prepare the assessment episode

■ Inability to 'twist the truth'

■ Developed the student's learning

■ Provided valuable feedback.

Portfolios used in a range of professions likewise had many positives, including the following:

■ Provided evidence of students' capabilities

■ Encouraged students as they could see their progress

■ Made students think

■ Gave them confidence

■ Were seen as a valuable method of recording feedback from people they had worked with

■ Were a useful reflective tool.

Other forms of practice assessment used in your own institution will likewise have many wider benefits beyond the grade awarded. Passmore and Chenery-Morris (2012) state that the combination of good mentorship, an assessment tool and grading should help students to progress. Try to use whatever methods your programme employs to help you develop as a student and future professional.

Pitfalls

Findings from the CEPPL study (Fisher et al. 2011) on the disadvantages of progress review *tripartites* included the following:

■ Difficult to arrange

■ Likened to a 'parents evening'

■ Found it challenging to express conflicting opinions

■ Verbal comments from sign-off mentor at the meeting did not always reflect previous feedback

■ Needed more feed-forward on how to improve as well as feedback.

The same study identified disadvantages of *observed assessments* as the following:

■ Could be difficult to arrange

■ Might need creativity to 'set up' the assessment which may not always reflect normal practice

■ Could lack authenticity due to the pre-planning and selection of the 'service-user' (woman) involved

■ The process of being observed could change the dynamics of the student–woman interaction.

Disadvantages of *portfolios* included the following:

■ Increased workload

■ Time-consuming

■ Needed forward-planning

■ Potential for breaching confidentiality.

Don't be disheartened by these 'pitfalls' but use your awareness of them to help you to work out ways of reducing or preventing them. Usually forward-planning and clear communication will do the trick. Don't be afraid to ask your sign-off mentor or academic assessor for additional feedback if they are not giving you sufficient information, and ask that they provide specific examples to help you understand where you may have been going wrong. Also ask them to provide you with specific guidance on how you can improve in the future. Remember that they are assessing your *performance* and not you as a *person* (though of course your personality may influence your performance), so try to take constructive criticism as just that. Some sign-off mentors may have the view that if they don't say anything it means you are doing fine – but it is important that they tell you this, so ask them for positive feedback too. If you are having any difficulties in your relationship with your sign-off mentor, please speak to your personal tutor, academic assessor or practice development midwife as soon as possible so that any issues can be addressed – a 'clearing the air' meeting will usually prove very helpful for everyone and will hopefully enable you to continue working together in a positive way.

Preparation

By now you must be feeling rather overwhelmed with the rules, regulations and terminology surrounding practice assessment, and perhaps a little anxious about the processes – although hopefully also seeing their benefits. It is not unusual for you to find it difficult to understand all these concepts prior to your first practice placement. Be reassured that everything will become clearer to you once you actually start using your practice assessment documentation and become familiar with the roles of those assessing you. It is also helpful to know some of the pitfalls you may encounter so that you can try to avoid them by careful planning and communication.

Box 3.4 provides you with some 'Top Tips' to prepare for your practice assessment. These prompts will hopefully guide you as you undertake your journey through your first and subsequent placements; you may wish to use them as a checklist. These 'Top Tips' are drawn from the longitudinal multiprofessional CEPPL study (Fisher et al. 2011) and are readily accessible as a booklet (CEPPL 2011) via the link in the 'Further Resources' section at the end of this chapter. If this link does not work, look for POPPI (Plymouth Online Practice Placement Information) through a search engine and the subsection on guidelines and policies in the 'Health' section. Note that there is also a checklist for staff on the reverse, so you can print this off and give your sign-off mentor a copy too. This booklet contains generic information which is suitable for any programmes with a placement focus.

Box 3.4 Top tips for preparing you for practice assessment

Before you go into practice (see also *Chapter 1*):

■ Review the feedback you have received in earlier placements and build on this in developing your learning objectives.

(continued)

- If you have a choice in your placement, ensure it will meet your leaning objectives and assessment requirements.

- Check out your placement – location, expectations, available learning opportunities, people to contact, dress code, transport and so on.

- Try to talk to previous or current students in this placement.

- Check that the placement is expecting you and that a designated sign-off mentor has been assigned to you as required by your programme.

- Visit or telephone the placement and introduce yourself to your sign-off mentor if possible.

- Check that the placement has the relevant current information about your programme and assessment (this is the University's responsibility to provide and the clinicians' responsibility to access, but there is no harm in you confirming this so that your assessment is up-to-date).

- Make sure you know who to contact for support if you have problems – both in the placement and University.

- Try to plan around competing demands, for example, practice and academic deadlines, personal commitments.

Early in your placement:

- Develop a learning contract in consultation with your sign-off mentor, based on your previous experience, the assessment requirements and the opportunities available in the placement.

- Set meeting dates with your sign-off mentor for regular feedback including a midpoint check on your progress and any summative assessments required.

Throughout the placement:

- Look out for and make best use of wider learning opportunities.

- Ask relevant questions and challenge practice appropriately to aid your learning.

- Be aware that your sign-off mentor has other demands on their time, and be flexible in your requests – remember that service-user needs take priority and your sign-off mentor also has a personal life.

- Obtain regular verbal and written feedback from a variety of sources, for example, service-users, other staff.

- Find out how you are doing and how you can improve – asking individuals to be specific in their feedback.

■ Clarify any questions you may have about your assessment criteria and documentation.

■ Keep all your practice documentation up to date including portfolios, timesheets etc – don't leave it all until the last minute!

■ Communicate any anxieties early and professionally to the appropriate person, for example, sign-off mentor, supervisor, personal tutor or other academic

■ Ask for support if you don't seem to be getting on with your sign-off mentor.

At your assessment point:

■ Plan meetings, observations or other assessments in good time.

■ Ask if there is anything you are unsure about.

■ Make sure your documentation reflects the practice learning you have achieved.

■ Obtain written reports from others as appropriate to support your evidence.

■ Be open and honest in documentation and discussions.

■ Accept the feedback given to you and make sure you understand the reasons for the judgement, asking for further information/clarification as needed.

■ Consider how to use the feedback constructively in identifying your future learning.

Source: Reproduced with permission of Centre for Excellence in Professional Placement Learning (2011) *Top Tips for Students: Your journey through Practice Assessment.*

Fitness to practise

This section is not meant to alarm you, but to raise awareness. It explains the Fitness to Practise (FtP) process which may, on occasions, be initiated if concerns are raised about a midwifery or nursing student's health or conduct which potentially compromises their status on the course or needs further investigation. The NMC requires a formal procedure to be in place in all higher education institutions providing professional programmes. This mirrors the Nursing and Midwifery Council's Fitness to Practise process which investigates allegations of a registered nurse or midwife falling foul of the NMC 'The Code' (2015). This recent professional publication has superseded the previous NMC 'Code' (2008b) and a specific booklet aimed at students: 'Guidance on professional conduct for nursing and midwifery students' (NMC 2011). You need to become very familiar with 'The Code' (NMC 2015) which comprises the standards expected of both students and registrants.

You may wonder why this subject has been included in Chapter 3. It may not appear on the surface that it relates to practice assessment. However, if you look back at the first section of the chapter in which the 'purpose' of practice assessment was discussed, you will see that it ensures that only safe, competent and professional students achieve registration as a midwife. To this end, you need to develop sound knowledge as well as demonstrate the appropriate skills, behaviour and attitudes in order to become a registered practitioner. If a personal or professional aspect of your performance is causing concern there is the potential for the FtP procedure to be invoked. This will result from a specific incident or series of events which appear to breach an aspect of 'The Code' (NMC 2015). Although the NMC (2011) publication aimed at students has been superseded by the above document, you may still find it helpful to refer to the specific examples of key aspects of students' clinical or academic performance or a personal behaviour which are inherent in the new 'The Code'. The following list is drawn from NMC (2011) pages 7 and 8:

■ **Aggressive, violent or threatening behaviour** (verbal, physical or mental abuse; assault, bullying, physical violence)

■ **Cheating or plagiarising** (cheating in examinations, coursework, clinical assessment or record books; forging a mentor or tutor's name or signature on clinical assessments or record books; passing off other people's work as your own)

■ **Criminal conviction or caution** (child abuse or any other abuse, child pornography, fraud, physical violence, possession of illegal substances, theft)

■ **Dishonesty** (fraudulent CVs, application forms or other documents; misrepresentation of qualifications)

■ **Drug or alcohol misuse** (alcohol consumption that affects work; dealing, possessing or misusing drugs; drink driving)

■ **Health concerns** (failure to seek medical treatment or other support where there is a risk of harm to other people; failure to recognise limits and abilities, or lack of insight into health concerns that may put other people at risk)

■ **Persistent inappropriate attitude or behaviour** (failure to accept and follow advice from your University or clinical placement provider; non-attendance – clinical and academic; poor application and failure to submit work; poor communication skills)

■ **Unprofessional behaviour** (breach of confidentiality; misuse of the internet and social networking sites; failure to keep appropriate professional or sexual boundaries; persistent rudeness to people, colleagues or others; unlawful discrimination)

■ **Criminal offences**.

You will see from this list that inappropriate use of social networking sites discussed in Chapter 1 would fall into this bracket; this is also specifically mentioned in standard 20.10 of 'The Code' (NMC 2015). This is a good example of what might be seen as a personal activity having a negative professional impact. Similarly, persistent failure to respond to constructive feedback and advice from your sign-off mentor or an academic could lead to invoking of the FtP process (also reflected in 'The Code', NMC 2015 in standards 9.2 and 22.3), or tampering with practice assessment documentation would constitute a breach of standard 10.3 – so you can see why it is relevant to this chapter.

Box 3.5 gives some real examples of issues which have caused concern and initiated an investigation in various programmes.

You will see from this list that some are clearly more serious than others. How far the FtP procedure progresses and the actions taken or penalties imposed will depend on this as well as the stage of the programme, the student's understanding and remorse and any contributory factors. Most stop at the early stages; very, very few would progress to the worst-case scenario which would be removal from the programme and inability to achieve the goal

---

Box 3.5 Examples of fitness to practise cases

- Inappropriate use of social networking sites

- Persistent non-attendance

- Timesheet discrepancies including fraudulent signatures

- Other fraudulent documentation, for example, sick notes, practice documents, extenuating circumstances forms

- Plagiarism

- Complaints from women or clinical staff

- Unsafe practice

- Drug errors or student administering drugs unsupervised

- Unprofessional behaviour

- Breaching confidentiality

- Breaching professional boundaries

- Inappropriate language

- Poor knowledge-base

- Aggressive behaviour

of becoming a midwife (in contrast to the worst outcome for a qualified practitioner which would be removal from the register and loss of a job). Students who are on a shortened programme as they are already on the NMC register as nurses need to be mindful that if a FtP investigation is conducted during their midwifery programme this may also impact on their nursing registration. You also need to remember that what you were able to do in a nursing post may no longer be applicable while you are a student midwife (e.g., your ability to administer medications without supervision), so be careful that you are very clear on your student status and professional boundaries.

Involvement in any stage of the FtP process is, of course, a very stressful time for the student (and those conducting the investigation). It is, however, an effective method of highlighting and addressing issues which – if they continued – could compromise a student's place on the programme or registration as a midwife, or worse still lead to a post-registration NMC FtP or supervisory investigation. Much learning can be gained from being involved – a lot depends on the student's attitude and the support offered during the process. Students generally become much more self-aware and appreciative of the true meaning of professional practice, which will hopefully result in a safer and more competent midwife who provides high standards of care.

I hope that you feel informed rather than frightened by this explanation. It emphasises the importance of professionalism in the career you have chosen, and your heightened awareness will hopefully prevent you going down this route in the future. Throughout this book you will see this concept reiterated, and the chapters on 'Introduction to midwifery and the profession' and 'What next?' put this into context.

Conclusion

This has been a very full chapter which has covered a range of topics around practice assessment and Fitness to Practise. It is hoped that you have found the information helpful in clarifying terminology and processes. You may find some aspects of your programme differ from the examples given; there are many roads leading to the 'Rome' of qualification as a midwife. The core principles will, however, be consistent across all institutions. Do join in any meetings or forums your Trust may provide in collaboration with your University to have a say in your practice placements and assessments. An excellent example is 'Bridging the Gap' – a meeting attended by clinicians, academics and students in one of the Trusts linked to Bournemouth University.

Use your practice assessment to be much more than a measure of your achievement of set criteria. See it as a developmental tool and a yardstick for your professionalism. Be creative and broad in your thinking about how best to gain the experiences needed. Keep at the forefront of your practice quality and the "6C's" (Department of Health 2012):

Care

Compassion

Communication

Commitment

Competence

Courage

- the outcomes and grades will then naturally be achieved.

To conclude with another quote from Georgia:

'It's easy to criticise yourself. Just remember how far you have come, and how much you know!'

References

Bower H, Fisher M, Jackson J, Chenery-Morris S (2014) Grading Practice in Midwifery Education: developing autonomous midwives for the future (presentation). International Confederation of Midwives 30th Triennial Congress, Prague.

Centre for Excellence in Professional Placement Learning (2011) *Top Tips for Students: Your journey through Practice Assessment.* Plymouth University, Plymouth. Available at https://www.plymouth.ac.uk/student-life/your-studies/academic-services/placements-and-workbased-learning/poppi/poppi-health/policies-procedures-and-guidelines (28 Feb. 2015).

Department of Health (2012) Compassion in practice: nursing, midwifery and care staff – our vision and strategy. Available at http://www.england.nhs.uk/wp-content/uploads/2012/12/compassion-in-practice.pdf (30 July 2014).

Duffy K (2004) *Failing students: a qualitative study of factors that influence the decisions regarding assessment of students' competence in practice.* Nursing and Midwifery Council, London.

English National Board for Nursing Midwifery and Health Visiting (2001) *Preparation of Mentors and Teachers.* English National Board, London.

Fisher M (2009) How can midwifery sign-off mentors be supported in their role? An evidence-based discussion of the challenges facing clinicians, managers and academics. *MIDIRS Midwifery Digest* 19 (3): 319–324.

Fisher M, Bower H, Chenery-Morris S, Jackson J, Way S (2015) An Exploration of the Application and Impact of Grading of Practice in Midwifery. *Nurse Education in Practice Special Issue: Celebrating Mentorship and Preceptorship in Contemporary Midwifery and Obstetric Nursing Practice* [under review].

Fisher M, Proctor-Childs T, Callaghan L, Stone A, Snell K, Craig L (2011) Assessment of Professional Practice: Perceptions and Principles. In: *Nursing Students and their Concerns.* (ed C.E. Wergers), pp 1–36, Nova Science Publishers, New York. Available at https://www.novapublishers.com/catalog/product_info.php?products_id=22965 (4 Aug. 2014).

Fisher M, Webb C (2008) What do midwifery mentors need? Priorities and impact of experience and qualification. *Learn Health Soc Care* 8 (1): 33–46.

Jervis A, Tilki M (2011) Why are nurse mentors failing to fail student nurses who do not meet clinical performance standards? *Br J Nurs* 20: 582–587.

Marsh S, Cooper K, Jordan G, Merrett S, Scammell J, Clark V (2015) Assessment of Students in Health and Social Care: Managing Failing Students in Practice. Making Practice Based Learning Work Project. Available at http://cw.routledge.com/textbooks/9780415537902/data/learning/5_Assessment%20of%20Students%20in%20Health%20and%20Social%20Care.pdf (28 Feb. 2015).

Nursing and Midwifery Council (2008a) *Standards to Support Learning and Assessment in*

Practice. Nursing and Midwifery Council, London. Available at http://www.nmc-uk.org/Documents/NMC-Publications/NMC-Standards-to-support-learning-assessment.pdf (1 Aug. 2014).

Nursing and Midwifery Council (2008b) *The Code: Standards of Conduct, Performance and Ethics for Nurses and Midwives*. Nursing and Midwifery Council, London. Available at http://www.nmc-uk.org/Documents/Standards/The-code-A4-20100406.pdf (28 Feb. 2015).

Nursing and Midwifery Council (2009) *Standards for Pre-registration Midwifery Education*. Nursing and Midwifery Council, London. Available at http://www.nmc-uk.org/Documents/NMC-Publications/nmcStandards forPre_RegistrationMidwiferyEducation.pdf (28 July 2014).

Nursing and Midwifery Council (2011) *Guidance on Professional Conduct for Nursing and Midwifery Students*. Nursing and Midwifery Council, London. Available at http://www.nmc-uk.org/Documents/NMC-Publications/NMC-Guidance-on-professional-conduct.pdf (4 Aug. 2014).

Nursing and Midwifery Council (2015) *The Code: Professional Standards of Practice and Behaviour for Nurses and Midwives*. Nursing and Midwifery Council, London. Available at http://www.nmc-uk.org/The-revised-Code/ (24 Feb. 2015).

Passmore H, Chenery-Morris S. (2012) Grading Pre-registration Midwifery Practice: A Concept Analysis. *Evid Based Midwifery* 10 (2): 57–63.

Rutkowski K (2007) Failure to fail: assessing nursing students' competence during practice placements. *Nurs Stand* 22: 35–40.

Further resources

Websites with useful frameworks eg: SWOT analysis/reflection models etc: http://www.businessballs.com/swotanalysisfreetemplate.htm.

Plymouth Online Practice Placement Information (POPPI): https://www.plymouth.ac.uk/student-life/your-studies/academic-services/placements-and-workbased-learning/poppi.

Chapter 4
LOW-RISK MIDWIFERY PLACEMENTS

Jo Coggins

Introduction

As a qualified midwife, your role will be to view pregnancy and childbirth as normal events and to be expert in providing support and care for women with uncomplicated pregnancies and births. Of all the practice areas you will experience throughout your training, there is arguably no better place to see this in action than during your 'low-risk' clinical placements. Depending on the structure of maternity services in your area of work, low-risk midwifery settings may take on a variety of forms. For example community-based midwifery teams, stand-alone midwife-led birth centres or co-located midwife-led birth centres. (These are birthing centres situated alongside acute maternity units but staffed only by midwives.) In some areas, maternity care is provided only within an acute unit and all women are cared for by the same team of midwives regardless of whether they have a straightforward or more complicated pregnancy. Each offers many learning opportunities and

here we will look at some of the ways you can prepare prior to entering placement to enhance your experience. Firstly, there are many professionals you may meet along the way; therefore, the following section provides a short overview of those you may meet and work alongside.

People you may meet

■ *Community mentor* will be your first point of contact during placement – a qualified mentor assigned to support and guide you in achieving your placement competencies and objectives. Make contact early if possible and discuss what you both expect from the placement. Be friendly and show your enthusiasm. Aim to work with her/him as much as possible as this will make it easier to follow your progress. Mid-way through discuss whether you both feel the placement is going well, including areas where you require more experience and create a plan to achieve this. Before leaving

The Hands-on Guide to Midwifery Placements, First Edition.
Edited by Luisa Cescutti-Butler and Margaret Fisher.
© 2016 John Wiley & Sons, Ltd. Published 2016 by John Wiley & Sons, Ltd.

meet again to reflect on the placement and to revisit the aims and objectives.

■ *Midwifery managers/clinical leads* are responsible for the day-to-day running of services, including staffing, budgeting, delegating workloads and doing appraisals. Try to spend a day shadowing the manager/lead for your area as it will give you an awareness of the complex issues affecting women's care that may not be so apparent otherwise, for example the wider political influences and financial constraints.

■ *Supervisors of midwives* (SOMs) are midwives appointed by the Local Supervising Authority (LSA) whose primary function is to protect the safety of mothers and babies. Currently, every midwife has an allocated SOM, although an official review in 2014 and published in 2015 called for a change in the law whereby supervision will no longer be statutory. It is expected that this change will take up to 2 years to come into force. The role of midwifery supervisors and midwifery supervision after this is not clear. In the interim, SOMs provide round the clock cover for women or midwives who wish to contact them. Every midwife has a SOM and in some areas you will be allocated a SOM who will oversee you throughout your time as a student. At Bournemouth University, for example, each cohort of students in every NHS Trust hospital where BU places students will have group supervision with their named SOM. Typically these meetings will take place three times in an academic year. If you don't know who your SOM is, please ensure to find out her/his name and their contact details. Also ensure you know how to contact the 'on-call' SOM when in practice.

■ *Specialist midwives* are those who are employed to focus on a specific area of practice or certain groups of women who may have particular needs. Examples include consultant midwives, practice development midwives, vulnerable adult midwives, teenage pregnancy midwives and so forth. Find out who the specialist midwives are in your area and what their field is. It may be helpful to arrange to shadow them for a day to learn more about what the role entails and how it benefits women.

■ *Obstetricians/ general practitioners* (GPs) share the care of pregnant women along with midwives in some areas whereas in other areas GPs have minimal involvement. Obstetricians are doctors with specific training to care for women during pregnancy and birth, particularly those with more complex medical needs. In the main, obstetricians work in larger maternity units and women referred to them by the community midwives go there for an appointment. Learn how women are referred and for what reasons. Local policies and guidelines usually contain this information.

■ *Maternity care assistants* (MCAs)/ *maternity support workers* (MSWs)/*auxiliary staff* whose role in maternity services has developed only in recent years. Like midwives, maternity care assistants (sometimes referred to as maternity support workers) have seen their role change a lot in recent years and they now play a big part in maternity services. Having successfully completed their training, they can perform many different duties depending on which setting they work in, although always under supervision from midwives. Experienced MCAs are an excellent source of knowledge and in low-risk settings they are often more involved with hands-on care of women, more so than those who work in larger units. They offer invaluable support to midwives and women and take on a wide range of duties such as taking women's observations, assisting women with breastfeeding and baby care and taking blood tests. Ask what the MCA's role and responsibilities are in your area. Working alongside MCAs is hugely important as a student in order for you to understand the working relationship between them and midwives and the important work they do. This will also help you feel more part of the team and them to feel their role is valued. Auxiliary staff are not trained to care for women in the same way as MCAs can and tend to be responsible for 'housekeeping' such as ordering stores, making up notes and information packs, restocking rooms and giving out food and drink at meal times.

■ *Volunteers/breastfeeding support workers* are often local people who volunteer their time to support women in birthing centres, sometimes doing 'tea rounds' or helping with making up information packs. Breastfeeding support workers have received training in breastfeeding and may also visit birthing centres to help women with feeding problems.

■ *Administrative assistants/secretaries/ward clerks* are arguably the mainstay of the smooth day-to-day running of a unit and frequently referred to as a 'font of all knowledge'! Responsible for all administrative and clerical requirements, they manage anything from requesting women's notes, arranging appointments, taking phone calls, overseeing electronic files and updating database information. They know the whereabouts of policies, procedures and protocols you may need to read, not to mention where to find equipment, how to contact outside agencies and who is responsible for what in the unit. Introduce yourself and don't be afraid to ask them if you are unsure of anything. If they don't have the answer, they will point you in the direction of someone who does!

■ *Health visitors* have close links with midwives in community units and often meet regularly to discuss care of women and families. If concerns are identified in pregnancy, the health visitor needs to be involved early on to help write a plan of care. Shadowing a health visitor is beneficial to help you understand what is in place for women once their community midwife has discharged them.

■ *Social workers* are those with whom midwives as part of their role in safeguarding are increasingly working in partnership. This might involve referral of women who require additional support at home, those who may need re-housing or women who have become victim to domestic abuse. In the event of safeguarding issues where midwives have concerns for the welfare of the unborn baby, early referral to a social worker and regular multi-agency meetings is crucial. The nature of this aspect of community midwifery can be both personally and professionally challenging but is necessary for the right and proper protection of women and babies.

Developing skills

Basic nursing care

Before your placement begins, remind yourself of the basic nursing skills you will need. These are the 'transferable skills' that are essential in any setting such as 'helping women with hygiene needs', remembering important infection control principles such as hand-washing and following manual handling guidelines. This way, as soon as you start, you will be able to offer basic care to women and get involved with some of the daily duties of the midwives. Figure 4.1 illustrates some of the basic nursing skills needed in low-risk midwifery settings. Don't think that these are 'mundane' or 'menial'. Maslow's hierarchy of needs clearly identifies the importance of these fundamental skills, and failure to meet them has resulted in recent hospital and care home scandals (e.g. the Francis and Keogh Reports) (Maslow 1943; Francis 2013; Keogh 2013).

Autonomy and leadership skills

As you near the later stages of training, it is an ideal time to begin thinking about how you will feel when you are working as a registered midwife. Being on placement in a low-risk setting lends itself to this as midwives in these areas are largely responsible for the day-to-day running of the service. Managing workloads, making decisions, working alongside other

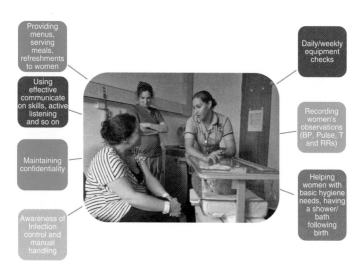

Providing menus, serving meals, refreshments to women

Using effective communicate on skills, active listening and so on

Maintaining confidentiality

Awareness of Infection control and manual handling

Daily/weekly equipment checks

Recording women's observations (BP, Pulse, T and RRs)

Helping women with basic hygiene needs, having a shower/ bath following birth

Figure 4.1 Basic nursing/midwifery care for women who are at low risk.

professionals and coping with staffing issues are all part of their role.

You can begin working more independently by asking your mentor to observe you whilst you do an antenatal or a postnatal check, and then discussing how you would go about supporting the woman if the decision was yours alone. Then build your confidence by following through a plan of care that involves, for example, referring the woman to a doctor or completing the paperwork to involve social workers in her care. This helps your understanding of the processes midwives become involved with and will develop your management skills. Ensure never to act without first discussing the situation with your mentor however. (See Chapter 5 where some of these skills will be mentioned in more detail and Chapter 6 where independent working can begin to be undertaken in conjunction with your community midwife.)

Managing the daily workload in a low-risk setting or taking responsibility of coordinating the team on shift in a birthing centre is also good for building on your leadership and management skills. You will need to think about the order in which you do things and how you divide up work between the staff. Of course, if a woman arrives in labour or someone phones in sick, you will then have to alter your plan! Ask your mentor to let you take the lead and make the decisions with her overseeing you.

In the same way that you practise 'drills' for clinical scenarios, ask your mentor to set scenarios to test your leadership and management skills. It will help to read up on different theories and also to watch the other midwives to see how they handle certain situations. Get into the habit of asking yourself; 'what would I do'? Remember your decisions should always be focussed around ensuring women receive the best possible care.

Before birth

Depending on the environment you are in, your daily duties will probably include a broad range of antenatal and postnatal care and also care of women in labour. Contact your mentor before starting to discuss some of the key tasks that you will be involved with on a day-to-day basis. These are some that you will likely encounter:

Pre-conception clinics

There is now greater focus on health promotion for women planning a pregnancy and pre-conception clinics are one way in which midwives are involved. They are usually quite informal 'drop-in' sessions in which women can come along and chat to midwives about ways to stay healthy when planning a pregnancy or in the early weeks after finding out they are pregnant. Revise relevant topics in order that you too can chat with women and offer advice. For example:

■ Current advice on diet and lifestyle changes when planning a pregnancy, including nutritional supplements such as folic acid and vitamin D (the NICE guidelines (NICE 2008) are a useful tool here).

■ Read up on the latest advice relating to women with complex social factors when trying to fall pregnant and during pregnancy.

■ Consider the effects certain medical conditions may have when women are trying to fall pregnant, such as diabetes or epilepsy, and whether women should be seeing their GP or specialist before becoming pregnant.

You will need good listening skills and remember to be sensitive to the fact that for many women planning a pregnancy and trying to get pregnant can be stressful. Any advice you offer should be up-to-date and in line with the Trust policies and guidelines. You can usually access these in the workplace or online but check with your mentor if you are unsure.

Booking Clinics

'Booking' is the term used to describe a woman's first appointment with her midwife. How and where this takes place varies. In some areas women are seen at home and in others it takes place in an antenatal clinic. Ensure to find out what the routine is in your area. At this stage, you will be completing women's maternity notes and the layout of these can vary greatly too. Get ahead by asking your mentor to send you a blank set before starting your placement, and familiarise yourself with them. This will save your time during appointments and will prevent any awkward moments when you are with women. As it is the woman's first appointment, there is often a lot of paperwork to complete or information to input to a database. Likewise, there are several issues to discuss and numerous tests to offer, and most importantly taking the

time to answer any questions she may have. Generally, the booking appointment includes the following:

■ Recording the woman's name, address, date of birth and next of kin details.

■ Confirming dates of her last menstrual period (LMP) and the probable due date for her baby (known as the 'estimated due date' or EDD).

■ Taking a thorough medical history (including partner and family) and identifying her risk of potential complications, that is developing conditions such as pre-eclampsia or gestational diabetes.

■ Referring women with increased risks to appropriate specialists, for example an obstetrician.

■ Taking and recording her blood pressure (BP).

■ Discussing and offering routine blood and urine tests such as those to confirm her blood group, iron levels and ruling out any urinary or vaginal infections. Testing for *human immunodeficiency virus* (HIV), hepatitis B, rubella immunity and syphilis are also commonly offered.

■ Discussing and offering tests relating to the baby's development (referred to as 'screening') which may include detailed scans, blood tests or more complex procedures.

■ Arranging routine scans, usually at 12 and 20 weeks.

■ Identifying whether the woman's social circumstances would require referral to social workers or to the local housing officer.

■ Considering the woman's mental health and whether she needs additional support.

■ Enquiring whether she is or has been exposed to domestic abuse (if this is an appropriate time/place to discuss such matters) and how to seek help if necessary, for example from women's aid or local refuges.

■ Considering any potential/current child protection concerns.

■ Arranging her follow-up appointments and ensuring she knows how to contact a midwife should she need to.

The sheer amount of information shared at this appointment can seem overwhelming. Try to adopt a methodical approach and use the maternity notes to prompt you. Remember also that whilst you are writing or typing, take time to make eye contact with the woman and to show her you are listening. It is widely known that important information can be gained from simply observing her body language or facial expressions. Community midwives play a key supportive role throughout women's pregnancies and it is important to establish a good relationship with women from early on.

Antenatal clinics

Working in antenatal clinics highlights the supportive role of community midwives and demonstrates the numerous clinical and non-clinical skills they need. In low-risk settings, clinics are midwife-led and there are often no doctors present. It is therefore important to be organised as appointments usually last only between 15 and 20 minutes. A typical appointment might begin with a general chat about how the woman is feeling and answering any questions she might have. Next step is moving on to the physical check-up which routinely involves taking her BP, testing her urine using a 'dipstick' and 'palpating' her abdomen to assess and measure the baby's growth and in the later stages of pregnancy to determine the baby's position (palpation is the term used to describe an examination using 'touch'). From around 12–13 weeks, you may also try to listen in to the baby's heartbeat using a Pinard stethoscope (a traditional tool used to listen to an unborn baby's heart) at first (as it is usually easier to hear with) and then with a 'doptone' machine so that the mother can hear it too (Fig. 4.2).

In late pregnancy, all women should be asked about their baby's movements as a decrease in the kicks she feels can sometimes suggest problems with either the baby or placenta. Whilst you are talking to her during the appointment, listen carefully for anything that may be concerning and ask yourself if she needs to be referred to other professionals. This might be health related requiring a consultant appointment or to do with her home situation, in which case involvement of a social worker may be needed. Current UK guidelines advise 10 antenatal checks for women who are considered low-risk and first-time mothers and just 8 for those who have given birth before (NICE 2010), so it is important to use this time wisely. Prepare well and find out how to refer women to

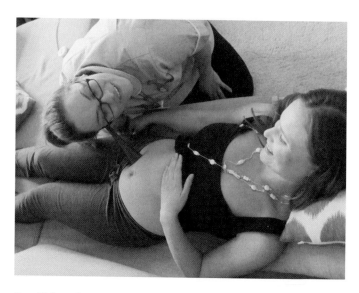

Figure 4.2 Using a Pinard stethoscope. A woman with her midwife at an antenatal appointment.

other professionals or organisations if necessary and how to input information to their electronic records if this is required. Also make a note of key phone numbers, such as those used to check blood results or to make appointments. Below is a handy checklist for use when working in a midwife-led antenatal clinic:

■ Ask the woman how she has been feeling lately and listen/look carefully to her reply.

■ Ask about life at home/work and whether there is anything that may affect her or her baby's health. Does she need referral to another specialist or organisation to help with this?

■ Review any previous test results, explain them to her and record them in her notes.

■ Record her BP and test her urine and record the results.

■ Discuss routine tests and take them if she consents, for example iron levels to check for anaemia and blood group/antibodies at around 28 weeks.

■ Check the baby's growth by measuring the height of the woman's uterus and feel for the baby's position (especially important in the last 4 weeks to check the baby is presenting 'head down').

- Listen in to the baby's heartbeat with a Pinard stethoscope and/or doptone machine and record the rate.

- Offer her any useful information that may help in her preparation for birth and motherhood, for example details of local antenatal classes including yoga/pilates/aquanatal sessions, information on breastfeeding and local support groups, and suggest a longer appointment at around 35 weeks to chat through her preferences for the birth.

- Ensure you have recorded details of the appointment in her notes and electronically if necessary.

- Check she knows how to contact a midwife routinely/out of hours.

- Arrange her next appointment.

Advising women over the telephone

Women should have round the clock access to advice in addition to their normal check-ups. Answering calls is something you can do early on in your training but check with your mentor first. Likewise, you should check your mentor is in agreement with any advice you give to women. Details of calls are usually recorded either in a diary or electronically; ensure you know what is done in your area. When speaking with women over the phone, remember the importance of confidentiality and do not give out information inappropriately. Finally, remember your NMC Code and be friendly, polite and helpful! If you are unable to help her, ask a midwife to come to the phone or take her number and arrange for someone to call her back.

Antenatal classes

Antenatal education is a routine part of antenatal care and is traditionally offered by midwives inviting women and their birth partners to come together as a group during late pregnancy to discuss issues surrounding labour and birth and adjusting to life with a new baby. Some areas also offer DVDs and online packages too. Organisations such as the National Childbirth Trust (NCT) also provide courses for would-be parents, although at a cost. Getting involved in antenatal classes is a great opportunity to develop your knowledge as they cover so many topics. Holding the class with your mentor is also good for your public speaking and presentation skills. Preparation is important and will calm your nerves. Here are some tips:

- Find out when and where the classes are held.

- Check the whereabouts of parking, toilet facilities and fire escapes.

- Discuss with your mentor exactly what your role will be during the class.

- Revise relevant topics, for example labour, pain relief and breastfeeding, and familiarise yourself with the local policies and guidelines.

- Encourage discussion within the group and group activities to help people get to know each other. You might want to bring along teaching aids to support your discussion, for example a model 'doll and pelvis' to demonstrate the baby's journey through the birth canal during labour or perhaps a DVD on breastfeeding.

■ Try to make the class fun, interactive and informative.

■ You might consider handing out feedback sheets to help you reflect and identify the things you did well and areas you can improve on for next time.

During birth

Care of women in labour

Looking after women in labour is often a really fulfilling part of your low-risk placement. In contrast to the fast pace and high-tech nature of a delivery suite, birth in a midwife-led unit (sometimes called a Birthing Centre) or in the woman's home is often a more gentle encounter and can leave you with a real sense of being 'with woman'. Before starting your placement, read around the topic of normal labour and birth. Use a wide range of resources to help you learn about the process of normal labour and how midwives can support women. The work of authors such as Balaskas (1994) and Gaskin (2002) offer particularly inspirational views on this and highlight the importance of helping women to view labour as a positive event and to work with their body's natural processes. Your care should be very 'hands-off' and focussed on encouraging women to remain active in labour, using upright positions to aid the baby's journey through the birth canal. Complementary methods (Fig. 4.3) for relieving pain such as hypnobirthing are used in low-risk settings (and sometimes in high-risk settings) and usually complement active labours and tend not to involve artificial drugs (see Table 4.1), although most birthing units keep 'gas and air' which is a mix of oxygen and nitrous oxide commonly known as 'Entonox'. Women typically inhale 'gas and air' through a mouthpiece or facemask during their contractions.

Accurate record-keeping when supporting women in labour is a very important part of a midwife's role and is in the Midwives Rules (NMC 2012). Explain the importance of record-keeping to the woman and her birth partner so that they understand what you are doing. Similarly, get to know your way around the paperwork so that you can record events accurately and swiftly. This will allow more time for you to be with the woman.

Birthing centres

There is much to consider when caring for a woman in labour in a birthing centre. Firstly, is it the safest option for her and the baby? For this, you will need to look at her notes to find out whether she has had a straightforward pregnancy. Ask her how she has been and whether there have been any complications. If she has had other children, ask how those pregnancies and births went too. In the main, women who choose to give birth in a birthing centre should be generally fit and well, but occasionally women with increased risks also opt for to go to a birthing centre. These women can be supported by offering them opportunity during their pregnancy to discuss their birth with their midwife and a Supervisor

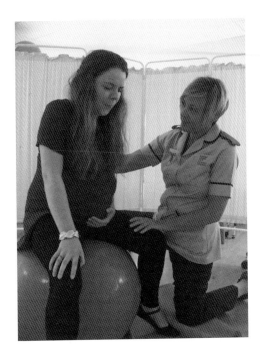

Figure 4.3 Woman in labour using a birthing ball.

of Midwives (see 'key professionals'). This means an appropriate plan of care can be put into place.

When caring for women in labour whilst in a birthing centre, the following are your key tasks and considerations:

■ Promote active birth principles such as encouragement to keep mobile and to be in an upright position for birth.

■ Consider the birth environment and maintain a calm and peaceful setting with plenty of space for the woman to move around.

■ Record her observations with minimal interruption to her and ensure they are within normal ranges, for example BP, temperature, respiratory rate and pulse.

■ When caring for her on arrival, you may decide whether it's necessary to examine her abdomen (palpation) for determining the position of the baby.

■ Explain the importance of listening to the baby's heartbeat regularly (every 15 minutes in the first stage of labour and every five during the second stage is

Table 4.1 Approaches to support women in labour.

Methods	How does it work?	Pros	Cons
Breathing/relaxation	Can help women feel more relaxed and at ease	No side effects and can be used with other methods	Women may need additional pain relief
Hypnosis (hypnobirthing)	Creates a deep state of relaxation	No side effects and can be used with other methods	Needs to be learnt and practised during pregnancy
Complementary therapies (aromatherapy, reflexology)	Uses massage and/or touch with scented oils to relax women	No side effects and can be used with other methods	Some oils are not advisable and reflexology can only be done by a trained person
Birthing ball	Balancing on the ball can reduce backache during labour	No side effects; excellent for helping women maintain upright posture to aid labour	Women may need additional methods alongside
Water	Takes the strain off women's bodies through floatation and enables relaxation	No side effects and can be used alongside some other methods; can relieve backache/pelvic pain	May not be available if hospital is busy; cannot be used with pain relieving drugs, for example, pethidine
TENS (transcutaneous electronic nerve stimulation)	Tiny electrical impulses delivered through a handset connected to pads on a woman's back. Interrupts pain messages to the brain and encourages release of body's natural painkillers (endorphins)	No side effects for baby; woman can control level; can remain mobile whilst using it	Cannot be used in water; needs to be used from early stages to get best results; may not be as helpful in later stages of labour

Table 4.1 (cont'd)

Methods	How does it work?	Pros	Cons
Gas and air (Entonox)	Mix of oxygen and nitrous oxide breathed through a mouthpiece or face mask	No side effects and can be used alongside other methods for baby; easy to use; wears off quickly	Can cause sickness; can give women a dry mouth
Pethidine/ diamorphine	Strong painkillers given by injection	Quick acting and strong painkiller; can help women to rest	Can cause sickness; can affect the baby – not advisable if birth is close

recommended) and do so with minimal interference to her.

■ Talk to her about events at home such as when the contractions started, whether membranes have ruptured and how often the baby has been moving. Observe her body language and offer to discuss some of the methods she could use to help make her more comfortable.

■ Ask yourself at regular intervals: Do I have any concerns for this woman or baby? Does she require medical attention and transfer to a hospital delivery suite? This is especially important in birthing centres located some distance away from the tertiary unit as even with a 999 ambulance transfer can still take a considerable time. Discuss any concerns promptly with your mentor and explain them sensitively to the woman so that she is fully informed. Always keep an accurate record of events.

■ Should the need arise to transfer the woman to a delivery suite, continue to encourage and reassure her. Getting into an ambulance whilst in labour can be very frightening for women and community midwives play a key role in supporting women having to do this.

■ Have a 'hands-off' approach. Remember that doing a vaginal exam (VE) should be one of the last skills used to determine a woman's progress during labour. If necessary, explain the procedure to her and pay close attention to her privacy and dignity (remember that abdominal palpation should always precede any VE). Wash your hands thoroughly and have your gloves to hand. *Wait* until she is ready and gently examine her vagina and cervix. Explain your findings and always use positive, reassuring language. In partnership with her and your mentor, agree a suitable plan of care and record this clearly in the notes.

■ For women in early labour, it may advisable for them to return home. Evidence points to better outcomes when women remain in their own surroundings for longer. That said, the decision should be made on a case-by-case basis and *always* in agreement with her. If she has a considerable journey to and from the unit or she has given birth quickly in the past, it is probably safer and more agreeable to her that she goes for a walk or sits in the relaxation area (most birthing centres have a quiet area for women to relax in during early labour).

■ If labour has established, you can show the woman to the birthing room and begin to agree a plan of care. Be led by her and consult with your mentor regularly. Ensure your practice is evidence based and your record-keeping is thorough. Facilitate her wishes and encourage her using lots of positive language. Create a calming birth environment; opt for subtle lighting, utilise birthing aids such as birthing balls or slings and put on some music if she wishes. Build a rapport with her and use your intuition to strike a balance between supporting her and reassuring her but also giving her privacy.

■ She may want to consider pain relief. Generally, birthing centres promote natural methods such as the use of water, birthing balls and aromatherapy or massage, although they often keep Entonox as this is a popular choice among women and has few side effects (see Table 4.1). Community midwives have a key role in supporting women during labour without the use of drugs. Take a holistic approach and involve her birth partner

with things like massage and visualisation. Supporting women through labour using these methods is not only a great learning opportunity to witness the physiology of birth when it is not interrupted by drugs but also the positive impact of one-to-one midwifery care that is not always available in delivery suite.

■ When preparing for the birth, as in any setting, ensure you have checked and prepared any equipment. In birthing centres, it is usual for emergency equipment to be stored outside the room so as not to disturb the birth environment.

■ Ensure you have means to summon help should complications arise and that your colleagues know the woman is soon to give birth.

■ As the baby is born, promote early bonding by placing her in her mother's arms as soon as possible and encouraging skin-to-skin contact. This is where the mother removes any clothing she may be wearing and holds the baby directly against her bare skin. It is known to promote bonding, encourage breastfeeding and helps to keep the baby warm.

■ A physiological birth of the placenta in which women push it out without the need for hands-on help from midwives is the norm in birthing centres, but some women can opt to have an injection known as 'oxytocic' which speeds this stage up by allowing midwives to gently pull on the umbilical cord to remove the placenta. The oxytocic is usually administered by an injection into a woman's upper thigh. The same principles of active birth offered during labour benefit women choosing to birth their placenta by themselves, for example upright postures, encouraging the woman to pass urine and ensuring she feels relaxed and unhurried. Early breastfeeding is highly recommended as this stimulates the hormone known as 'oxytocin' which stimulates contractions that give women the urge to push the placenta out (Baker 2013).

■ Another advantage of breastfeeding soon after the birth (if this is the woman's preferred method of feeding) is that it often leads to more successful breastfeeding once the woman has gone home. The 'baby check' can wait until the baby has been fed and can be done whilst she is in her mother's arms. Weighing isn't urgent and can be left until later. These first moments between a mother and her baby are precious and should not be rushed.

Homebirth

Supporting women choosing to birth at home can be a wonderful experience and is a great learning opportunity. Aim to read key articles/research relating to homebirth such as those produced by the Birthplace in England Collaborative Group (2011), anthropologist Sheila Kitzinger (2002) and Wesson (2006). To be involved with homebirth you will need to be 'on call' with your mentor, so ensure she has a means of contacting you. Each unit or team will have equipment specifically for homebirths, so try to familiarise yourself with this when first starting. It's also a good idea to check the whereabouts of any women due to give birth whilst you are on placement to ensure you know how to find them. You should not go into the woman's home alone and should always meet up with your mentor first. Homebirth requires the same key midwifery skills you would use when supporting any woman in labour but in an environment in which you may not be so familiar. To ensure both the woman and her midwives are kept safe, it is normal practice to complete a 'homebirth checklist' in the final weeks of the woman's pregnancy. This includes things such as whether there is easy access to the house, if there is sufficient space and lighting and whether there is a phone line or signal in order to call a second midwife for the birth or ambulance should complications arise.

Here are some important points to remember when caring for women at home:

■ Consider your lone working guidelines and ensure someone in the team or unit knows where you are and how to contact you. Do not enter the woman's home alone.

■ Remember you are a guest in her home. Be respectful of her possessions and her cultural preferences.

■ Remain quiet and calm allowing her to focus. Discussions between midwives should take place quietly and phones should be set to vibrate/silent.

■ When listening in to the baby's heartbeat, do so without distracting her if possible. Use a Pinard's stethoscope or doptone depending on her position and always reassure her after listening.

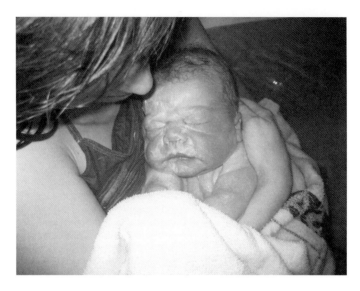

Figure 4.4 A woman and her baby experiencing skin-to-skin contact following a water birth.

■ Involve her birth partners or family members including children or pets (!) as is her choice and remember this is a special time. Respect their privacy.

■ If she asks for pain relief, encourage natural methods such as relaxing in a bath or listening to music. Partners can help by giving a massage. Gas and air (Entonox) is usually available to women birthing at home too.

■ Remember your NMC Code and be friendly but professional.

■ Work with her and facilitate her choices where possible but also consider safety for her, her baby, you and your mentors.

■ Perform any physical examinations sensitively and regard her privacy.

■ If transfer to hospital is necessary, the reasons why need to be carefully explained to the woman. She may feel less anxious if she knows what is likely to happen when she gets to the hospital.

■ As the baby is born, place her into the woman's arms for skin-to-skin contact and encourage early breastfeeding (Fig. 4.4).

■ Encourage the woman to birth her placenta naturally and advise her on the things that can aid this (see 'Care in Labour: Birthing Centres')

■ Respect this special time for her and her family. Do not rush to carry out routine checks. Respect her privacy and consider writing your notes in another room to give her and her new family some time together.

■ When the time comes to leave, ensure she knows how to contact a midwife if necessary. Arrange for a midwife to visit her later that day or tomorrow. See Vignette 4.1 which describes Lauren's first experience of a low risk placement allocation.

Care of women who are at low risk in high-risk areas

Your low-risk placements will not necessarily be in the community or in a birthing centre. You may be placed in a large 'delivery suite' set within a maternity unit. These are often extremely busy as they provide care for large numbers of women, particularly those with medical problems and those with complications in pregnancy. Obstetricians and midwives work together in these settings but there is generally a more 'medicalised' approach

---

Vignette 4.1   A students eye view

When preparing for my first low-risk placement, I felt feelings of excitement at the idea of going out and working with women and being able to put the theory I had learnt into practice. It's also normal to feel nervous and the first few days of a placement can seem overwhelming. During the early stages of your training, try not to panic and feel you have to learn everything at once. You will have opportunities throughout your course to put your learning into practice, so be patient with yourself.

My placement was in a midwife-led birthing centre and I really enjoyed being able to consolidate my understanding of normal pregnancy and practising key skills such as listening to fetal hearts using a Pinard, performing abdominal palpations and taking women's baseline observations. Being able to spend time with women and chatting to them whilst undertaking checks was also very rewarding. There is widespread evidence that one of the key attributes midwives need is to be able to listen actively, taking on board women's fears and concerns and being able to address them with empathy and compassion. However, I discovered early on that although the midwives did their best to dedicate time to every woman they saw, at times their workload made it almost impossible. Consequently, whilst my mentor was arranging appointments or completing entries on the computer, I would sit and chat with women. This is where I felt I was really able to make a difference and my mentor agreed it was a good use of my time, as it built on my existing knowledge and generally gave me greater insight into women's needs and expectations. Talking to women about their experiences is a key learning opportunity when on placement and is something I now aim to do as much as possible.

In the first few weeks I was quite overwhelmed, not to mention exhausted, by how much there was to learn. So many abbreviations to take in, written records

---

to learn, computer systems to navigate, policies to read and people to get to know. But, half way through I began to develop confidence in myself and in my own abilities. I was completing palpations and vaginal examinations and understanding what I was feeling and with each birth I felt happier about my normal midwifery skills and began to broaden my knowledge of supporting women in low-risk settings, in particular the use of non-pharmacological methods of pain relief in labour. I felt that I started to become useful by helping to write notes and finish the computer work after births, as well as talking to and supporting women whether they were in antenatal clinic, during labour or postnatally if they needed help with breastfeeding and baby care.

Reflecting on my first few shifts, there are numerous things I would advise fellow students to do: When preparing for placement, not only minimise your own stress but also make the most of the learning opportunities on offer to you and 'fit in' with the team:

■ Ensure you have all the contact numbers that you need – the placement area number, a contact number on which you can reach your mentor and a number to contact your University should you need to call in sick.

■ Ensure you know your mentors name, your visiting lecturer for your placement area (sometimes called a Practice Area Link Midwife or 'PALM') and your personal tutor should you need any support whilst on placement.

■ Ensure you know the shift pattern and times and your off duty for the first week.

■ Check the car parking policy. See whether you will need to pay, do you need to get a parking permit and what to do if there is little parking.

■ Check the uniform policy paying close attention to footwear, ID badges and wearing of jewellery and see if you need to buy scrubs or whether these are provided.

■ Think about carrying a notebook with you as it can be really useful to make notes of things to remember when in new placement areas. You will encounter a lot of information in the first few shifts and jotting things down may make life easier.

■ Ensure you have a supply of black and red pens for record-keeping. The NMC requires that we keep clear and accurate records of the care we provide.

■ Be open to learning as much as you possibly can. Don't be afraid to ask questions but ensure to ask them at appropriate times. If necessary, use your notebook so that you can remember to ask the question later. Discretion is the key as a student midwife!

■ Ensure you have revised your 'normal ranges', including blood pressure ranges, fundal heights and fetal heart rates, as well as signs and symptoms of early pregnancy and tips to help with things such as morning sickness. Read up on issues specific to low-risk care; promoting active birth, physiological third stage and facilitating water birth/home birth.

■ Don't panic and remember your mentor is there to guide you.

I see placements as a crucial step along the journey to becoming a midwife and being in a low-risk setting gave me fantastic insight into truly 'normal' midwifery. I was glad I had prepared well prior to starting as this allowed me to settle in quickly and alleviated (some of) my anxiety. I worked hard and seized any opportunity to develop my skills or broaden my knowledge. As a result, I feel better equipped to enter the next stage of my training.

Lauren Orchard
Ex-student, University of West of England, Bristol

to care in comparison to the more natural processes seen in birthing centres. There are still many women who for one reason or another go to a delivery suite to give birth even though they have few risks. When caring for these women, you should use the same skills and methods you would use when caring for a woman at home or in a birthing centre. It is often easy to resort to medical intervention such as the use of epidurals or unnecessary use of equipment such as electronic monitors to listen to the baby's heartbeat simply because they are to hand (see Chapter 5 for more information on these settings).

After birth

Postnatal care

As is the nature of modern maternity services, women's postnatal care tends to vary from place to place. Ask your mentor how women are supported in your placement area. Some Birthing Centres offer inpatient stays for

breastfeeding support, whereas some do not. Similarly, some midwifery teams visit women at home whilst in other areas women come to 'postnatal clinics'. The care and support midwives give in the early weeks following their birth is hugely important to women and can help prevent complications such as painful breastfeeding or postnatal depression. Postnatal care covers a wide range of issues for women and babies and advises changes regularly as new research is done. Ensure you update yourself prior to entering your placement to be confident that the care and advice you give is the best it can be. The following are the main areas in which midwives can offer women support (Fig. 4.5):

■ Offering basic nursing care immediately following the birth, for example helping women to freshen up, get changed and to have refreshments.

■ Offering regular pain relief to those women who have had complicated vaginal births or caesarean sections.

Women's first midwife appointment: 'Booking'

Antenatal checks of women and their unborn babies

Using national guidelines to care for women with low-risk pregnancies

Recognising and referring women and babies with complications

Promoting healthy lifestyle choices for women before, during and after pregnancy and childbirth

Drop-in clinics, for example pre-conception clinics, breastfeeding support groups

Helping during antenatal classes/preparation for birth

Advising women over the telephone

Working in community teams

Record-keeping: accurately recording care and advice given to women

Breastfeeding support

Postnatal care of women and their babies

Supporting women through labour and birth using natural methods of pain relief

Caring for women in labour in birthing centre or at home including waterbirth

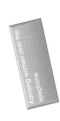

Figure 4.5 Key tasks.

- Carrying out daily checks on women and their babies, answering questions and performing routine tests such as BP, pulse and temperature for women and the heel-prick test for babies. Each check should also include discussion about how the woman is feeling emotionally.

- Getting medical help for women or babies who develop complications.

- Offering help and advice on breast-feeding and explaining the benefits for mothers and babies.

- Respecting that some women choose to artificial feed and supporting them equally.

- Performing checks to see that the mother's body is recovering well, for example feeling her abdomen to check her uterus is returning to its normal size and asking if her toilet habits are normal.

- Recognising women who are showing signs of depression and offering additional support such as more frequent home visits or referral to their GP or Health Visitor. This is a really important part of women's postnatal care and can have long-term consequences for women if it is not handled well.

- Undertaking the examination of the newborn. This is usually done at around 24 hours following the birth and is a thorough 'head-to-toe' examination. It used to be performed by doctors on the postnatal wards but now it is undertaken by many midwives after extra training and can be done in women's homes, in postnatal clinics or on the ward.

- Advising on all aspects of baby care, including feeding and encouraging healthy development, bathing, skin care, sleeping and observing for signs of illness.

- Offering opportunity for women to reflect on their experience of pregnancy, birth and the transition to family life, including the care they have received. Women's feedback is hugely important not only for their future physical and emotional health but also to improve the service midwives provide.

- Arranging women's discharge from midwifery care and discussing issues relating to their ongoing health and well-being, for example resuming smear tests, arranging a 6 week mother and baby check with the GP and considering contraception if desired.

Dos and don'ts for community working

Community midwifery by virtue of the name involves caring for women and families in their homes. In contrast to the formal, rather clinical setting of a hospital or surgery, being able to engage with women in their own homes can be particularly rewarding and can encourage good relationships between midwives and women. That said, it is also important to recognise the potential risks involved with this way of working. It's likely as a student you will carry out visits with your mentor but it is never too early to consider ways in which you can not only protect the women in your care but also you and your colleagues.

Uniforms

- *Do* check the local uniform policy and follow it.

- *Do* ensure your uniform is clean and presentable.

- *Do* ensure your ID badge is visible at all times.

- *Don't* wear your uniform to/from work (most units provide laundry services and changing facilities).

- *Do ensure* that – if uniform is not worn – your personal clothing is clean and professional. Avoid low-cut tops, figure-hugging trousers and bare midriffs!

Being with families in their homes

- *Do* remember to be polite and respectful, for example removing shoes when entering/switching mobile phones to vibrate.

- *Do* carry drinks/snacks if you will be in the house any length of time, for example during a homebirth.

- *Do* remember health and safety and infection control measures, for example hand-washing.

- *Do* carry out a risk assessment if the woman is planning a homebirth.

- *Do* consider whether the environment is safe and suitable, think about space, access, safety and hygiene.

- *Do* follow the lone-working policy if you are undertaking visits under indirect supervision later in your programme.

- *Do* remember your equipment and ensure it is working properly.

- *Do* note the nearest exit should you need to leave quickly.

- *Don't* forget record-keeping in the woman's notes and in your work diary (this is a legal document).

- *Don't* forget confidentiality. Consider what you say and who is present during your visit – it may be appropriate to ask the woman if she would like friends/relatives to go to another room whilst you are there. See Box 4.1 which has more top tips for you: before you start, during and finally after completion of your low risk placement allocation.

Box 4.1 Top Tips

Before starting your placement:

- Make contact with your mentor to introduce yourself and clarify where and when to meet on your first shift. (*Tip*: It can be a little tricky to get hold of your mentor, so leave yourself plenty of time! Don't phone in the first half an hour of a shift as handover will be taking place and your mentor may not be able to talk!).

■ You may not be able to get all your shifts for the whole placement before you start, so try and be flexible.

■ Ensure you have the correct uniform and shoes ready for placement.

■ Read through you paperwork and competency documentation thoroughly and ensure you clearly identify what you need to achieve during your placement.

■ Chat with other student midwives in the cohorts above you, you will gain lots of insights and tips from them.

■ Ensure you know where you are going, where you can park before your first shift and leave yourself plenty of time to get there!

■ Revise your mechanisms of normal birth and read up on water birth and home birth.

During your placement:

■ Familiarise yourself with the placement area, this will make you feel more comfortable and confident if you can find things when needed. Your mentor will give you a tour on your first shift.

■ Ask questions and seek feedback on your progress and development from your mentor.

■ Recognise your limitations and ask for support when needed. You are a student and you are learning; you will not know everything straight away!

■ Create a learning plan with your mentor and discuss with her what you need to achieve during your placement. Review this through the placement to ensure you are on track!

■ If you have any difficulties, seek support. This could be from your mentor, another midwife or your personal tutor at University.

■ Remember from your first shift you will be working and supporting women and their families. Ensure you act professionally at all times, you are representing your University, your placement area and midwifery!

■ Remember your code and confidentiality as to what you can share with friends and family about your shifts.

■ Catch up with others in your cohort, but try not to compare yourself against them. Every student gains different experiences at different times.

■ Smile and be enthusiastic!

■ Work hard and enjoy yourself!

(continued)

When your placement has finished:

■ Reflect on the experience you have gained during your placement; this includes the highs and the lows.

■ Review your feedback from your mentor, the areas of competency you have achieved and your areas of development identified for your next placement.

■ Use events that happened during placement to act as a trigger for further reading and research.

■ Meet with your personal tutor to discuss your placement. Seek support if you need it.

■ Look forward to your next placement!!

Rachel Pass
Ex-student, University of West of England, Bristol

Conclusion

This chapter has introduced you to low-risk midwifery and the opportunities available to you whilst in placement. It has outlined the healthcare professionals you will meet and the skills you can develop and enhance whilst working with women who are low-risk. In addition perspectives and key learning opportunities are provided for working within the community and the hospital environment. Finally the chapter concludes with student viewpoints including a vignette by Chelsea (4.2) which explores her experience of being on shift one night and the magic of being with a woman during her labour and birth.

Vignette 4.2   The sun will always rise tomorrow

I'm standing upon a precipice and darkness is enveloping me. Wave upon wave crashes against me, systematically exploiting my weaknesses, leaving me weary. The murky fog rolls in, clouding my vision and perception, leaving me scared to take a step forward in case that step plunges me deep into the abyss. I don't know what to do. I grasp out for something, not knowing what but still I grasp. The anxiety wells up inside me, paralysing me and I can no longer think coherently. Cortisol is flowing through my veins, and my shoulders slump and my head throbs. I feel like crying. I feel like screaming. I want to curl into a ball and hibernate. Fight or flight; fight or flight. I don't know which to do. I want to fight but sometimes flight seems easier. No, I must fight. I take a step forward and another step. I am wading through some opaque and viscous substance and each step requires insurmountable energy and courage. No wonder I feel so tired but onwards I go for I don't want to look back tomorrow and think I could have done more.

Just when I feel like the night will never end upon the horizon, I see the first whispers of dawn as the sun ascends tantalisingly and begins illuminating all before

---

me. As my vision comes back into focus, I remember the moments of achievement. The first time I did a baby check and the sense of euphoria and achievement that beseeched me. The wonderment of palpating a baby and being able to determine its position and correctly diagnosing a breech baby. These moments collate themselves to form a sense of identity and notion that you are a student midwife.

The morning bursts into recognition and the night begins to fade into the distance. The breeze is bracing and I feel refreshed. I had coped with the moments thrust into, like the day I turned up at the children's centre and there was no midwife to work with. Instead I helped facilitate a parent education class. The anxiety of the night dissipated and I thoroughly enjoyed myself. I felt the radiance and power of the sun beat down upon me instilling a confidence. The women who ran the class said that I had made a difference and the class had never been so participative.

As the sun reaches its pinnacle and there are no shadows and the cascading rays of sun brighten and glisten. The time is golden and I recall the first baby I saw come into the world. It was an experience that I will never forget. The women clicked her fingers through each contraction. I remember thinking 'oh now what do I do' when the midwife left the room, but all I had to do was remind the woman to breathe through her contractions. The power of nature took over and everything man-made forgotten. All that mattered were this woman and her baby. I remember the satisfaction I felt when the partner said 'you'll make a good midwife'. After the little girl was born, the family wanted a photo of me and insisted that I have a photo for my memories.

I remember my most precious and sacred moments with clarity. The parent's reactions when their child is born, whether they are thanking god for their gift or tears are rolling down their cheeks and falling upon their babies head christening it with love. It is their wide eyes ready to take in the sight of their precious baby that will always be etched upon my memory. It is at that moment when I see them become a family and you remember just how much this moment should be treasured and honoured.

The shadows begin to lengthen as the sun descends and in the twilight I reflect on the things that make my job unique. The impact you have upon families lingers past dusk and into the nights and days to follow. The father who is too scared to hold his baby but tentatively helps me to dress her and peers into her cot and watches her sleep. The 16 year old who feels reassured by my presence as I pop up unexpectedly at a parent education class, on labour ward and in clinic. I see her grow from a girl who cannot answer questions for herself, always relying on her mum to a young woman who can talk in front of a group of people at a parent education class.

As the sun begins to set once more, I don't worry for I know the sun will always rise tomorrow.

Chelsea Butchers
First-year student, Bournemouth University, Dorset, UK
Reproduced with permission of Chelsea Butchers

References

Baker K (2013) How to promote a physiological third stage of labour. *Midwives* 16 (5): 36–37. Available at http://www.rcm.org.uk/midwivesmagazine/features.

Birthplace in England Collaborative Group (2011) Perinatal and maternal outcomes by planned place of birth for healthy women with low risk pregnancies: the Birthplace in England national prospective cohort study. *BMJ* 343: d7400.

Francis R (2013) *The Mid Staffordshire: Report of the Mid Staffordshire NHS Foundation Trust Public Enquiry.* The Stationary Office, London.

Kitzinger S (2002) *Birth Your Way.* Dorling Kindersley, London.

Keogh B (2013) Review into the quality of care and treatment provided by 14 hospital Trusts in England: overview report. Available at http://www.nhs.uk/NHSEngland/bruce-keogh-review/Documents/outcomes/keogh-review-final-report.pdf (last accessed 9 September 2014).

Maslow AH (1943) A theory of human motivation. *Psychol Rev* 50: 370–396.

National Institute of Clinical Excellence (2008) Pathway: routine care of all pregnant women. Available at http://www.pathways.nice.org.uk (last accessed 12 March 2014).

National Institute of Clinical Excellence (2010) Clinical Guideline 62: Antenatal Care – routine care for healthy pregnant women. Available at http://www.publications.nice.org.uk (last accessed 12 March 2014).

Nursing Midwifery Council (2012) Guidelines for records and record keeping. Available at http://www.nmc-uk.org (last accessed 12 March 2014).

Useful reading

Balaskas J (1994) *New Active Birth: The New Approach to Giving Birth Naturally.* Harvard Common Press.

Gaskin IM (2002) *Spiritual Midwifery*, 4th edition. Book Publishing Company.

Kitzinger S (2002) *Birth Your Way.* Dorling Kindersley, London.

Royal College of Midwives (2012) Evidence based guidelines for midwifery-led care in labour. Available at http://www.rcm.org.uk (last accessed 17 March 2014).

Royal College of Midwives (2014a) i-Learn: women, families and society. Available at http://www.ilearn.rcm.org.uk (last accessed 19 March 2014).

Royal College of Midwives (2014b) i-Learn: lone working – advice and good practice. Available at http://www.ilearn.rcm.org.uk (last accessed 19 March 2014).

Wesson N (2006) *Home Birth: A Practical Guide.* Pinter & Martin Ltd. Available at http://www.aims.org.uk/pubs.htm (last accessed 4 March 2015).

Further resources

http://www.activebirthcentre.com.
http://www.rcm.org.uk.
http://www.nmc-uk.org.
http://www.nice.org.uk.
http://www.nct.org.uk.
http://www.independentmidwives.org.

Chapter 5
HIGH-RISK MIDWIFERY PLACEMENTS

Margaret Fisher

Introduction

Midwives are the experts in normality in the childbearing continuum. We do our best to promote this at every opportunity, and try to work in partnership with women to achieve normal childbirth as far as possible. The International Confederation of Midwives (ICM) Position Statement on 'Keeping Birth Normal' (ICM 2008, p1) supports the following definition:

> 'A unique dynamic process in which fetal and maternal physiologies and psychosocial contexts interact (with the goal of mother and baby being well). Normal birth is where the woman commences, continues and completes labour with the infant being born spontaneously at term, with cephalic birth presentation, without any surgical, medical or pharmaceutical intervention, but with the possibility of referral when needed.'

At times, however, things do not go according to plan and physiology may turn into pathophysiology. Women may embark on a pregnancy with existing psychological, medical, physical or social problems. Women or babies may develop complications during the journey. These deviations from the normal can affect the care required – and indeed the outcome itself. It is these situations which may be deemed 'high risk'. But does this mean that midwives no longer have a role to play? Does it mean that *all* the care the women or their babies will require will be in the realms of 'high risk'? Does it mean their needs will bear no resemblance to those of women who are at low risk? Does it mean that the outcome will inevitably be abnormal?

The answer to all the questions above is a resounding 'No'! Midwives have perhaps an even greater role to play in that – while remaining vigilant and responding in a timely manner to any problems – we need to help the women *feel* as 'normal' as possible, and promote this at every opportunity. We need to try to keep the rest of their pregnancy, labour and postnatal period as low key as we can – not forgetting important aspects such as parent education and breastfeeding support in the midst of what may otherwise be a very medicalised experience. For example, there is no

The Hands-on Guide to Midwifery Placements, First Edition.
Edited by Luisa Cescutti-Butler and Margaret Fisher.
© 2016 John Wiley & Sons, Ltd. Published 2016 by John Wiley & Sons, Ltd.

reason why women cannot be encouraged to be mobile in labour within the constraints of any monitoring and interventions. Mothers still need information, support and reassurance. They may need us even more as their advocate. We need to be true partners in their care.

Caring for women and neonates at high risk therefore requires midwives to demonstrate a range of skills, a depth of knowledge and a woman-centred attitude. It is for this reason that high-risk midwifery placements will be extremely valuable as you will witness for yourselves, and gradually begin to participate in the care of these women who perhaps need their midwife even more. This chapter seeks to prepare you for placements which – although challenging – can help you to function effectively in this role.

Learning opportunities available

Clinical areas to which you are allocated will vary in what 'high-risk' situations may present. At one end of the scale, you may be placed in low-risk settings such as community and stand-alone, midwife-led or alongside birth centres. At the other end, you may be allocated to an acute, specialist maternity unit in which 'high risk' is bread and butter to the staff. Somewhere in between you may be placed in maternity units which cater for women and babies who are in low and medium risk categories, having the

facilities to cope with deviations within certain constraints before they may require tertiary referral to a more specialised hospital. These may include, for example, maternity units which will accommodate women after a certain gestation (e.g. 29 weeks) – prior to which they would have been under the care of a centre with more specialist neonatal facilities. The following categorisation of neonatal care was introduced in the United Kingdom in 2011 by the British Association of Perinatal Medicine (2011):

■ *Intensive care:* Care provided for babies who are the most unwell or unstable and have the greatest needs in relation to staff skills and staff to patient ratios.

■ *High dependency care:* Care provided for babies who require highly skilled staff but where the ratio of nurse to patient is less than intensive care.

■ *Special care:* Care provided for babies who require additional care delivered by the neonatal service but do not require either intensive or high dependency care.

■ *Transitional care:* Care that can be delivered in two service models, within a dedicated transitional care ward or within a postnatal ward. In either case, the mother must be resident with her baby and provide care.

Wherever you are placed, it is important to remember that 'low risk' can quickly turn into 'high risk' and vigilance is therefore needed throughout the period you provide care to women and their babies. Emergencies can occur

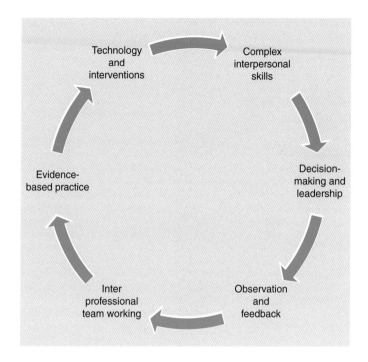

Figure 5.1 Learning opportunities in high-risk areas.

in any setting, and you can learn a great deal from these experiences (Fig. 5.1).

Learning through observation and feedback

If you have the opportunity to care for someone who is deemed to be at 'high risk', there is valuable learning to be gained. Rather than being frightened by the prospect, keep your eyes and ears open, ask questions and read around the situations and conditions you may encounter. Although you may have already developed the skills needed in caring for women who are at low risk and becoming increasingly independent in this practice, you are likely to be more directly supervised when encountering 'high-risk' care. Take advantage of this – not only to learn from what you observe and from responses to your questioning, but also from the opportunity of the midwife (or other professional) working more closely with you to provide feedback on how you are performing. It is common for first-year students to experience direct supervision for much of their practice, thereby learning from the role-modelling of other practitioners whilst gaining valuable feedback on their own performance. As your programme progresses, you will find that you work more independently and are expected to practise under decreasing levels of supervision. Although this is as it should be and prepares you for the autonomous role of the midwife, it means that opportunities to either watch other professionals or gain feedback on your own directly observed practice become rarer – so make the most of these. You will also benefit hugely from observing others' practice when you already have some knowledge and experience under your belt, picking up valuable tips and examples of different ways of doing or saying things. See this closer supervision when caring for women in high-risk settings as a really positive opportunity for learning.

Learning from the interprofessional team

An important aspect of caring for women in high-risk categories is interprofessional teamwork. The fact that complications exist means that the midwife must refer mothers or their babies to appropriate professionals or agencies, and not work in isolation. This requirement is clearly stated in the 'Midwives Rules and Standards' (NMC 2012, Rule 5, Standard 4, p 7):

> 'In an emergency, or where a deviation from the norm, which is outside of your current scope of practice, becomes apparent in a woman or baby during childbirth, you must call such health or social care professionals as may reasonably be expected to have the necessary skills and experience to assist you in the provision of care.'

As midwives, we work in both multiprofessional and interprofessional teams. In multiprofessional working, many professionals from the same or different backgrounds work in a united team to achieve a common goal or purpose (e.g. in an emergency situation). However, we also work interprofessionally – as distinct but collaborative professions or agencies within the common care environment – each contributing our own knowledge, skills and support. An example would be the care of a pregnant woman with complex social and physical needs, when each individual or agency has a specific function to perform. For the purposes of this chapter and other relevant sections in the book, the term 'interprofessional' will be used – particularly in the context of the care environment.

A co-ordinated approach to care is one of the main messages in the recent 'Mothers and Babies: Reducing Risk through Audits and Confidential Enquiries across the UK' report (MBRRACE-UK 2014) – failure to do so contributing to a number of the maternal direct and indirect deaths included in this document. This need for teamwork is also emphasised in 'The Code' which requires registrants (and therefore also students) to *Work cooperatively* (NMC 2015, Standard 8, p 8).

You will encounter a range of professionals, agencies and support workers in the context of your high-risk placements:

- Obstetricians

- Anaesthetists

- Operating Department Practitioners

- Paediatricians or Neonatologists

- Neonatal nurses

- Physiotherapists

- Dieticians

- Social workers

- Health visitors

- Physicians and surgeons

- Specialist midwives or teams (e.g. substance misuse, domestic abuse, perinatal mental health, infection control), tissue viability

- Psychiatrists

- Ultrasonographers

- Haemotologists

- Theatre and recovery nurses

- Maternity Support Workers/Care Assistants

- Porters

- Laboratory staff

- Paramedics

- Pharmacists

This list is far from exhaustive, but gives you a picture of the huge network of professionals and support staff which may be needed in the care of just one woman. Teamwork is therefore crucial, and communication paramount. You will find it very valuable to spend time shadowing some of the individuals above as you will gain a clearer understanding of what their role entails; it will also help you to feel and be seen as a part of the team. You may have this opportunity while undertaking your high-risk placement, or it may be more appropriate to focus this learning in specific periods of your programme when more choice may be possible (see Chapter 7 for further information). Take full advantage of every opportunity you have to observe and discuss these differing roles and how they fit into the care pathway and jigsaw of holistic care of the woman or baby in whose journey you are involved.

Remember that teamwork is not all a question of you 'taking' the learning, but also you 'giving' to the individuals in that team. Be responsive to call bells and requests for assistance, offer help if you see someone struggling or you do not have another task to do at the time, join in making the beds when the area is busy and make cups of tea for your colleagues to help keep them sustained. You will find yourself welcomed into the team, you will feel useful and you will also gain additional learning opportunities by being proactive in putting yourself out for others. Don't just take it from me – look at some of the comments from students in their vignettes and the 'Top Tips' section of this and other chapters.

Learning about evidence-based practice

Throughout your programme you will be learning the underpinning theory at University and in your wider reading, and applying this to the context of your practice settings. Your high-risk placements will provide you with wonderful opportunities to expand your knowledge base. You will gain a real appreciation of the importance of guidelines, policies and protocols in informing practice. You will learn the importance of robust evidence being used to devise these documents and processes. You will see real-life application of international and national guidance and the importance of adhering to this in order to provide safe and consistent care. You may also witness the professional response to situations in which decisions may not be clear-cut, and flexibility and adaptation may be needed within appropriate boundaries and following consultation with relevant practitioners such as the supervisor of midwives (SOM). All of this will build on your existing knowledge base, making you a safer and better practitioner in the future and enabling you to provide women and their partners with informed choice.

Standard 6 of 'The Code' (NMC 2015, p7) states that registrants (and students) must

> 'Always practise in line with the best available evidence'.

Lifelong learning

You will also discover that all professionals are constantly learning, and exchange of experiences and knowledge can be a fascinating and invaluable resource. You may well find that you can contribute to this by sharing some of the recent evidence you may have learned about in University; mentors often say that the experience of supporting students is a two-way learning process. I well remember working alongside a student midwife while engaging in clinical practice as a lecturer and encountering her 'hands-off the perineum' approach to helping a woman birth her baby. Having never seen it before and being a product of midwifery training in the 1980s in which a very 'hands-on' approach was the norm, I questioned the student on her rationale and she shared with me what she had learned from her mentor. I went and read up about the then recently published 'HOOP trial' (McCandlish et al. 1998) and changed my own practice thereafter, becoming much more considerate of whether or not any physical involvement in supporting the head or perineum was needed on an individual basis.

Skills and drills

You may also have the opportunity of attending in-house 'skills and drills' sessions when in a high-risk placement – do take full advantage of any opportunities, and be proactive in volunteering to be a 'patient' as you will learn a lot by listening to the professional discussions while you are at the receiving end.

Guidelines and policies

You will find some useful websites at the end of this chapter which comprise 'Position Statements', evidence-based guidelines and systematic reviews of the research. Textbooks such as the PROMPT manual (Winter et al. 2012) will also be valuable adjuncts to your learning. Use these in conjunction with your local Trust policies and guidelines to better understand the management of a range of high-risk conditions and emergency situations. You will find that if you spend time asking questions and reading up around experiences you encounter, you will be able to link theory with practice and vice versa much better. That exam question or OSCE (Objective Structured Clinical Examination) station you face in the future will be much more meaningful as you recall a practice experience and how it was managed. Most importantly, you will be able to draw on these experiences in future practice and have a clearer understanding of your own and others' roles – see Vignette 5.1 for Eloise Fanning's reflection on shoulder dystocia as an example.

Vignette 5.1 Shoulder dystocia learning

'During a shift on labour ward as a first-year student midwife, I was caring for a multiparous woman who was at low risk. She had been in the birthing pool since her cervix was 5 cm dilated and after a long first stage of labour her cervix progressed to full dilatation and the woman started pushing involuntarily. After an hour and seeing no signs of progression during the second stage of labour, my mentor decided it would be best for the woman to get out of the birthing pool to assess the situation. On examination the vertex was visible, so I prepared for the birth and used the call bell for a second midwife.

As the head delivered, the face was only visible to the nose and the head was tightly applied to the vulva and retracting. With the next contraction, there was no further descent or any restitution and the head started "turtle necking". This is when the fetal shoulder, most likely the anterior shoulder, impacts on the symphysis pubis. I pressed the emergency alarm bell as instructed by my mentor.

Before help arrived, we laid the woman flat and hyper-flexed her legs into McRoberts position as this opens up the pelvis to the largest diameter, and we discouraged the woman from pushing. As help arrived, my mentor stated that the emergency was a "shoulder dystocia" and the consultant obstetrician and his team took control and performed manoeuvres whilst I kept the couple calm. I tried to explain to them what was happening even though this was the first time that I had observed an obstetric emergency. The second midwife documented times and procedures performed and my mentor gave the woman's history to the neonatal team. After what seemed like hours, which were in fact minutes later, the baby was born in poor condition. My role was to stay with the couple whilst the neonatal team performed life support on the couple's son.

Having never experienced a shoulder dystocia before, it was traumatic and unexpected but I didn't have any other emergency to compare it to. Thankfully, the baby went home well after several weeks on the neonatal unit.

(continued)

Since this experience, I cared for another woman with no risk factors in my third year who had a shoulder dystocia. I was more confident, recognising the signs much earlier and I was clear of everyone's roles in the room and this was obvious as my autonomy had increased. I was able to document the times, manoeuvres and the health professionals present; this gave me great satisfaction as I was able to use the skills that I had learnt from my experience in the first year.

Learning

■ When an emergency situation arises again in my midwifery training or as a qualified midwife, I will continue to support the woman but I would take the leadership role.

■ I believe you learn a great deal from University but to actually witness, experience and learn from an emergency in a real-life situation is invaluable.

■ I am going to develop my own folder of local Trust guidelines and familiarise myself with the different risk factors for emergencies, and ask to spend time with my SOM to audit notes that I have documented as accurate record-keeping supports the care provided.

■ I have been told by my mentor that if an emergency arises, it is always good practice once you are home to write a reflection after the event as not only does it help you to personally debrief but it may also be useful if the family decide to take legal action in years to come. You can then refer to your own personal statement of the event which helps you to remember the details in more depth.

■ If I had another emergency where I felt that I would need to debrief, I would also discuss the event with my SOM to not only escalate the experience but to get an experienced midwife's view compared with my own view as a preceptee.'

Eloise Fanning
Third-year student, Plymouth University, Devon, UK
Reproduced with permission of Eloise Fanning

Learning about technology and interventions

Because of the 'deviation from normality' in high-risk placements and emergency situations, opportunities for extending your knowledge and skills in relation to technology, procedures and pharmacology will greatly increase. Intervention will inevitably be needed, and along with this will come experience not only of the equipment, products, policies and protocols but also of the decision-making around how much and when to intervene. Make good use of these opportunities, watch, ask questions and participate under appropriate levels of supervision and within local guidelines.

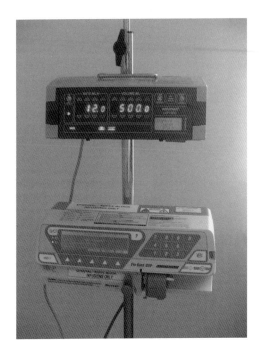

Figure 5.2 Intravenous and epidural pumps.

The following are some of the examples of technology, equipment, procedures and medicines you may encounter in your high-risk placements (Fig. 5.2):

■ Cardiotocograph (CTG)

■ Intravenous infusions (IV) and associated administration sets and pumps

■ Epidurals

■ Urinary catheters

■ Fetal blood sampling

■ Instrumental deliveries, for example forceps or ventouse

■ Episiotomy and perineal suturing

■ Caesarean section and post-operative care

■ Other operative procedures such as manual removal of the placenta or hysterectomy

■ Emergency procedures, e.g. management of cord prolapse, shoulder dystocia, ante or postpartum haemorrhage, maternal collapse, eclamptic seizure and neonatal resuscitation

■ Patient Group Directives, Midwives Exemptions and Prescription Drugs and Protocols (ensure you follow the current NMC guidelines – NMC 2007 'Standards for Medicines Management' at the time of publication).

Many mnemonics or algorithms exist to help professionals remember actions to take in emergencies or facilitate following of procedures. Check your local policies, professional websites or textbooks or of course draw on your University lectures. Share any particularly useful ones with your student peers and professional colleagues.

Learning about more complex interpersonal and communication skills

'Communication' is one of the essential skill clusters for midwifery (NMC 2009a) and threads through all the others; the range of skills you will need to demonstrate in a variety of situations will keep you busy. Nicholls and Webb (2006) found that communication was an essential element of a 'good midwife' – and this is particularly important in high-risk situations.

Communication with women and their families

You may face particularly challenging interpersonal encounters due to language barriers, cultural differences and social or mental health issues. You will see women who are frightened, confused, overwhelmed and feel out of control of their environment and their own bodies. You will encounter partners and family members who may demonstrate anger, frustration and high levels of anxiety. Verbal communication as well as behaviour may be volatile and intense. Keep professional at all times and seek help if needed. Watch and listen – you will learn much about how to communicate effectively through observing others in a range of complex situations. Rachael Callan, previous student at Bournemouth University, bears witness to the value of this in an excerpt from a reflection in Vignette 5.2. Your midwifery programme will include theoretical

---

Vignette 5.2 Interpersonal skills

'I feel one of the good aspects of this experience was that I managed to control my own emotions and remain professional, which was something I was not sure I could do. I also feel that watching the way my mentor dealt with the situation and listening to what she was saying to the couple was a very positive experience. I now feel that I have some idea of how to cope with emotional situations like that. I think it was good that the couple just had time and freedom to say whatever they wanted, and it was good that we were not telling them anything about how they should feel or saying we know how they felt when really we had no idea.'

Rachael Callan
Previous midwifery student, Bournemouth University, Dorset, UK
Reproduced with permission of Rachael Callan.

---

preparation for dealing with challenging situations and developing the necessary interpersonal skills; ensure you read up relevant lecture notes and texts as well as attend any available in-house training.

Interprofessional communication

Not only do communication and interpersonal skills need to be enhanced in your encounters with the women and families in your care, but you also need to develop appropriate professional interactions. These will include verbal, non-verbal and written communication. The extensive list of other professionals and support workers who may be involved in a woman's care was discussed earlier in this chapter. You can see why clear communication is therefore essential. You will need to brush up on correct terminology and develop the art of being succinct but informative, especially in your hand-over or reports to colleagues in the interprofessional team.

Learning about decision-making and leadership

The value of learning around decision-making you will experience in high-risk settings cannot be underestimated. In order to develop the skills required of an autonomous practitioner of the future, it is essential that you find out more about how and why decisions are made. Risk assessment and management are part and parcel of this role. Working with other members of the interprofessional team, experiencing a range of clinical situations and being involved in emergencies will all help you to be exposed to decision-making and

leadership. Take the opportunity – especially in your final year – to work with ward managers and co-ordinators; you will see things from a different perspective and gain valuable experience. This is discussed further in the section that follows which details learning in specific placement areas.

Ask practitioners how they reached certain decisions – but do this with the attitude of 'I'm a student and I want to learn from your experience' rather than in a challenging way which may not receive such a positive response. You will learn much from them. Sometimes the result will be that professionals question their own practice, which can make for positive changes.

Sharing your own thinking around situations and suggesting appropriate actions to take is a vital part of demonstrating your increasing competence which will reassure the sign-off mentor assessing you of your ability to perform as a future autonomous practitioner. Decision-making and leadership skills are essential in midwifery, and the more experience you gain through observation, discussion and your own activities while a student, the better prepared you will feel at point of qualification. A study undertaken in the United Kingdom (Skirton et al. 2012), known as the 'MINT study', identified reduced levels of confidence and experience felt by many newly qualified midwives in the area of high-risk care such as obstetric emergencies. Time management and multitasking were seen as gaps, particularly in busy postnatal wards. By gaining as much experience as possible in these areas of work as a student and developing your knowledge base and decision-making skills to support your practice, you will find the transition to qualified midwife a less stressful experience. See Chapter 9 which goes into further details about the importance of this approach.

In summary, *key learning* to be obtained from these placements includes the following:

■ Witnessing and learning from others' practice and interpersonal communications.

■ Gaining feedback on your own performance.

■ Learning about the roles of other members of the multidisciplinary team.

■ Developing your teamworking skills.

■ Experiencing in practice what you have been taught in theory, enhancing the links and your own understanding.

■ Learning what can go wrong and how to deal with it.

■ Developing more specialised skills and knowledge.

■ Increasing your awareness and implementation of policies, protocols and guidelines.

■ Increasing your knowledge of evidence-based practice.

■ Developing your decision-making and leadership skills.

■ Learning how others respond in stressful circumstances, and developing your own coping strategies and communication skills.

■ Gaining a greater appreciation of the lived experience of women whose situation deviates from the normal – learning about their anxieties, fears and concerns and the impact on them and their families.

■ Increasing your sensitivity and intuition so that you will be better able to pick up 'vibes' in your future practice.

Types of high-risk placements

So where are you going to learn all of these new skills and develop your confidence and competence in high-risk care? As part of your programme, you will almost certainly have at least one placement in each area listed in Fig. 5.3.

In these placements you will find that the midwives work much more closely with other members of the inter-professional team. You will also find that the locations seem busier, more stressful and confusing when you are new to them. Some students (and midwives) get a real 'buzz' from these environments, whilst others feel more in their comfort zone in home or other community settings and on postnatal wards. In order to register as a midwife, it is essential that you develop the skills to work safely across the range of clinical areas. It is therefore important that you approach each of these placements in a positive frame of mind and plan your learning so that you can achieve the required competencies and make best use of the opportunities available.

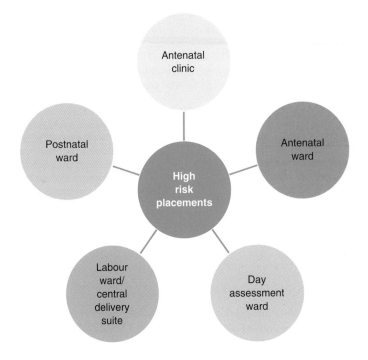

Figure 5.3 Types of high-risk placements.

A short explanation about each of these placements now follows, together with some examples of the learning you can expect to gain in each.

Antenatal clinic

In line with the National Institute for Health and Clinical Excellence (2011) 'Antenatal Care Pathway', the women you encounter in a hospital antenatal clinic will be requiring additional care to that routinely provided for pregnant women. They will therefore have needed referral from the 'low-risk' midwife-led care, and be requiring input from a wider interprofessional team. This will usually mean that the rest of their pregnancy and labour will be consultant-led – although on occasions women may initially be referred to a consultant clinic but then be able to return to midwife-led care for the remainder of their pregnancy. In practice, care is generally shared – and although input from the consultant or registrar is needed on one or more occasions in pregnancy, much of the care in the antenatal and labour periods may be provided by the midwife, with referral to a doctor as required.

The hospital antenatal clinic will therefore provide you with valuable learning:

■ *An excellent opportunity for you to observe, listen and learn* about complications or conditions and their management.

■ *Shadowing the consultant* so that you can learn more about their role and decision-making about the care the woman and her unborn baby will need in a range of situations. Most consultants will be very receptive to a student working with them, enjoying teaching and imparting their knowledge.

■ *Follow a woman through her antenatal care pathway.* If possible (and with her consent as well as permission from the midwife or doctor with whom you are working) accompany her for any blood tests, scans or other investigations as well as attend the clinic appointment itself. She may also be having a consultation with another health professional, so again try to accompany her to this. These experiences will provide you with a more holistic understanding of what management her condition or complication requires, and also the opportunity to meet and work alongside other members of the interprofessional team.

Antenatal ward

This is a valuable opportunity for learning about deviations from normal physiology, monitoring and interventions. You may also benefit from continuity of providing care which will be satisfying for both you and the women. Try to gain a holistic picture of the woman and her condition. Spend time asking her what her experiences have been to date, participate as fully in her care as you can, listen to discussions between the members of the interprofessional team and read her case notes. Read up guidelines and policies and compare these with the care you have seen being given. Supplement your experiences with reading around the conditions or interventions.

Women who are on the antenatal ward may well have anxieties about their own and their unborn baby's well-being, be worried about children back at home and be missing the contact and support of their families. They and their partners may therefore demonstrate a range of emotions. You may also come across a variety of psychosocial situations, and other members of the interprofessional team may be contributing to the women's care such as social workers, drug keyworkers or specialist midwives. Use these opportunities for learning more about the complexities of backgrounds of the women you encounter so that you may be better prepared for future situations.

The following are some of the examples of reasons for women being on the antenatal ward:

■ Monitoring of an unborn baby or pregnancy 'at risk' such as intra-uterine growth restriction, preterm pre-labour rupture of membranes, preterm labour, antepartum haemorrhage, multiple pregnancy or unstable lie.

Monitoring of a maternal condition such as diabetes or hypertension (raised blood pressure) which may be pre-existing or caused by the pregnancy such as pre-eclampsia or HELLP syndrome.

■ Treatment of infections.

■ Induction of labour.

Day assessment unit

Most acute maternity units will have a day facility for antenatal care. Women may self-refer (e.g. with reduced fetal movements), be referred by a community midwife from a clinic or the home setting (e.g. with hypertension) or be referred by a doctor from the hospital antenatal clinic or antenatal ward (e.g. for further investigations). In most cases, these units are staffed by midwives who have received further training, and they are able to undertake a number of investigations without needing to refer to obstetricians or other health professionals unless there are concerns. They also work closely with the wider inter-professional team in caring for women with more complex needs. You will have the opportunity to witness – and perhaps participate in – some of the more technological investigations.

Key learning in this placement will include the following:

■ Risk assessment and decision-making.

■ 'Triage' skills.

■ Referral pathways.

■ Interprofessional liaison and team-working.

■ Technological skills, for example ultrasound scanning, Doppler studies and amniotic fluid assessment, amniocentesis and chorionic villus biopsy.

■ Counselling skills, for example antenatal screening tests such as Down's syndrome, haemoglobinopathies and other genetic disorders.

■ Perinatal mental health and substance misuse.

■ Following of policies and care pathways, for example management of reduced fetal movements, glucose tolerance tests, pre-eclampsia monitoring, monitoring of the intra-uterine growth-restricted fetus and preparation for elective caesarean section.

These units are often extremely busy and there is high-throughput of women. Staff will therefore value your teamworking and you too will feel glad you have a role to play in undertaking some of the more basic procedures. The care will inevitably be one-to-one, and this again offers you excellent opportunities to learn from both the staff and the women. You will also find that the knowledge gained in this placement will inform the explanations you are able to give women in the future when you are in other antenatal settings – whether low or high risk.

Labour ward or central delivery suite

Along with the routine low-risk labour care explained in Chapter 4, you will gain a wide range of additional experiences and skills in this high-risk environment

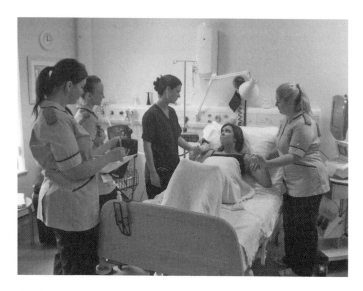

Figure 5.4 High-risk labour ward.

(Fig. 5.4). You may initially find some of these alarming or overwhelming, but stay close to the midwife with whom you are working and you will gradually increase your knowledge and confidence through questioning, observing and participating. Remember that the woman, her fetus/baby and family need to remain central to your care. If you think it is an alarming setting for you, how much more so for them? Don't underestimate the value of your support, providing a familiar face and voice in what may be a frightening time for them. The midwife you are working with will also value your assistance and team-playing, so use your initiative in helping out – fetching equipment, making

telephone calls, writing contemporaneous records and answering bells are just a few examples. You will also be exposed to numerous occasions of decision-making and referral activities – watch and listen and (at an appropriate time) follow up with questions and further explanation about anything you have not understood. Learn about teamworking, use of technology, the identification of deviations from the normal and how to manage these.

Emergency situations

You may well encounter emergency situations while in a labour ward placement. Try to keep calm and focused.

Observe, listen and work within the team. As your knowledge and skills develop through exposure to this setting, the theoretical information gained at University and your wider reading and asking of questions, you will find that you are able to play more of a part in these incidents. Try to debrief with the midwife or doctor with whom you have been working in order to better understand what happened, why this occurred and how a similar situation could be identified, prevented and managed in the future. Read up policies and guidelines and relevant literature to reinforce your learning. Millie Westwood, third-year student, describes an incident which demonstrates that you need to be prepared to 'expect the unexpected' in Vignette 5.3:

Vignette 5.3   Expect the unexpected

'I met Fiona whilst working a night shift on labour ward. Her labour was induced because of a prolonged rupture of membranes . . . Fiona's labour progressed well after the syntocinon infusion was started; her partner was very supportive, rubbing her lower back and giving her words of encouragement. I remained in the room for 2 hours, monitoring her contractions and CTG trace, offering my support when needed by reassuring her and suggesting new coping mechanisms to use.

[. . . I had been taking a break when I was called] by a flustered midwife telling me to get ready as we had to go to theatre with Fiona for a category two emergency caesarean. The midwife hurriedly mentioned that Fiona was bleeding and that blood clots had been noticed. I immediately panicked; had I missed something vital during my monitoring of Fiona? I knew that I had reported all findings to my mentor, and that she had also often been in the room, but I was terrified that I had missed something crucial and that I had caused this emergency. Holding back my emotions, I entered the room and took control of collecting the paperwork whilst midwives bustled around Fiona preparing her for theatre. I had no time to find out what had happened – Fiona and her baby were the priority, and we had to act quickly.

. . . The obstetrician who had performed the caesarean subsequently came to talk to Fiona . . . and explained to her that she had a bicornuate uterus, and that her placenta had started to separate which led to her bleeding during labour – a complication that could neither have been predicted nor rectified. I also learnt that the bleeding had started when her forewaters had been artificially ruptured by the midwife who had taken over when I was on my break. I felt instantly relieved that I had not missed any signs, and happy for Fiona that she had an explanation as to why she [had needed a caesarean section].

(continued)

'. . . There is a vast amount to learn as a student midwife, and this was a fraught but interesting case. I realise that I, and perhaps many qualified midwives too, may always automatically feel a sense of internal panic that something vital may have been missed when an unforeseen emergency arises during labour, even if one is confident that all observations have been done conscientiously.'

Millie Westwood
Third-year student, Bournemouth University, Dorset, UK
Reproduced with permission of Millie Westwood

Record-keeping

Record-keeping will form a major part of your learning in a busy labour ward. You will realise the importance of maintaining contemporaneous notes and learn the skill of including the relevant information. You will also discover a range of new documents and proformas. Computer records will also provide a steep learning curve. Try to get as involved as you can in documentation, and ensure you develop a practice of always writing down what you have done. Don't forget that all your entries must be checked and counter-signed by the midwife with whom you are working, whether this is under direct or indirect supervision. Follow the guidelines on record-keeping in 'The Code' and 'Midwives Rules and Standards' (NMC 2015, 2012) as well as the specific guidance in 'Record Keeping: Guidance for Nurses and Midwives' (NMC 2009b).

Co-ordination of the labour ward

Try to spend some time working with the co-ordinator towards the latter stages of your programme; you will learn valuable skills of prioritising, delegation, decision-making, problem-solving and management such as ordering of drugs, equipment repair and co-ordination of activities of the various members of the interprofessional team. You will also gain a better understanding of the complexities of care in a busy labour ward and be exposed to a range of experiences as the co-ordinator responds to calls for assistance and advice.

Perinatal death

On occasions, you may encounter the care of a woman undergoing late termination of pregnancy, an intra-uterine death or stillbirth. These are of course very challenging and emotional experiences for not only the woman and her partner but also the staff caring for her. It is suggested that you embrace any opportunity you may have to be involved, in a sensitive and considered fashion. The needs and wishes of the woman and her family must remain paramount, but if she consents to your involvement it is hugely beneficial for you to experience this aspect of high-risk care while you have the direct support of a midwife. It is likely that the midwife will also value your support, so again use your teamwork and interpersonal skills to contribute positively

Vignette 5.4   The art of silence

'Having discussed the experience with my mentor after it happened and having read around the subject of silence, I now realise that silence is not something to be afraid of but should be embraced as an effective communication skill and a tool for building a therapeutic relationship with a woman. Most importantly, I have learnt that women may actually respond better to silence than to me trying to comfort them with words. I have learnt that women need time to reflect themselves and I should give them time to do that without making them feel uncomfortable or rushed. However, I have not sufficiently developed my ability to deal with silence yet. I still need to work on my own attitude towards silence and focus on adjusting my body language in those situations so that I am not displaying my feelings of awkwardness or making the atmosphere tense. I need to learn to accept silence and embrace it rather than follow my initial instinct to avoid it. This skill will be useful to me as a midwife because I will be able to support women better as I will be encouraging their own reflection and allowing them the time to say whatever they feel they need to. I will not be overpowering them and dominating the interaction in order to fulfil my own needs, which will improve my relationship with the woman and I will be of more use to her.'

Rachael Callan
Previous midwifery student, Bournemouth University, Dorset, UK
Reproduced with permission of Rachael Callan.

to the situation. Ensure you have the opportunity to debrief and reflect on the experience after the event. Although Rachael wrote Vignette 5.4 as part of a reflection on a baby with abnormalities, the same principles are very appropriate to the context of caring for a couple who are experiencing bereavement; the art of silence cannot be underestimated.

Informed consent

Timely and appropriate explanations at a level she understands are vital to the woman's emotional well-being; ensure you know the correct information or listen to the midwife or doctor as they explain. Make sure her consent is

obtained and decisions are informed. 'The Code' (NMC 2015) is specific in this requirement in Standard 4.2 which states that we must

> 'make sure that you get properly informed consent and document it before carrying out any action' (p 6).

Standard 1.3 which discusses the need to

> 'avoid making assumptions and recognise diversity and individual choice' (p 4)

as well as Standard 2 which states that we must

> 'listen to people and respond to their preferences and concerns' (p 4)

and communicate clearly, using

'terms that people in your care, colleagues and the public can understand' (Standard 7.1, p 7).

Promoting normality

Very importantly, hold onto the concept discussed in the introduction to this chapter – that the role of the midwife is to promote normality where possible, even when some aspects of care have needed to become more medicalised. Keep in mind the 'basics' such as encouraging the woman to be as mobile as possible in her labour. What positions could the woman feasibly adopt while an intravenous infusion is running and her unborn baby is being continuously monitored on a cardiotocograph (CTG)? Does she need to stay on the bed or could she sit on a chair or birthing ball? Ensure that the woman is kept hydrated and comfortable; again the 'basics' can help enormously such as a cool cloth for wiping her face, regular changing of contaminated bed linen, frequent alternation of position when her mobility is more limited with an epidural and offers of a mouthwash or facilities to brush her teeth if she is unable to eat or drink. Involve the partner or birthing companion as they too will feel out of their comfort zone and may find the situation easier if they are able to participate in rubbing the woman's back, wiping her face or offering drinks.

Look after yourself

Take breaks when you can and make sure you always come supplied with snacks and drinks to keep your energy levels up. Remember that you must *always* inform the midwife you are working with if you are leaving the woman or labour ward; it is a busy place and essential that the co-ordinator is able to locate all staff (including students) at all times.

Key learning to be gained in this placement includes the following:

■ Care and monitoring of the woman and her unborn baby during high-risk labour.

■ Observation or participation in interventions such as induction of labour, epidurals, intravenous therapy, fetal blood sampling, instrumental or assisted delivery, and caesarean section.

■ Experience of obstetric and neonatal emergency situations and the associated teamworking.

■ Care of women experiencing intrauterine death, late termination of pregnancy and stillbirth.

■ Policies, guidelines and protocols.

■ Medicines management.

■ Record-keeping.

Postnatal ward

Much of the care provided to the new mother and her baby on the postnatal ward will reflect that seen in Chapter 4. For many women in high-risk categories, the most stressful times of the antenatal period and labour will be over, but for some these will only just be starting. Although many activities may be routine, it is very important to keep the individual woman at the centre of your care and adapt procedures and explanations to her needs. Try to work around her and her baby's timing where at all possible – this is not always easy in a busy postnatal ward, but needs to be considered. Many women will be very tired after a long labour which may have included a number of interventions, and it is important that they are able to rest as much as possible. Likewise, their babies may be exhausted, have a headache and be finding the adaptation to their new environment challenging, so treat them gently and patiently. The noise of other activities and babies crying will probably be contributing to stress and tiredness for both. Support in feeding – whether breast or bottle – will also greatly contribute to mother and baby satisfaction and sleep, so it is worth spending time assisting in this.

Key learning will include the following:

■ *Clinical skills*: Post-operative observations, urinary catheters, wound drains, intravenous therapy, wound care, suture removal and medicines administration. You may wish to include these 'nursing' skills as learning objectives in any non-maternity opportunities (see Chapter 7 for further information).

■ *Examination of the newborn*: Shadow these midwives (or neonatologists/paediatricians if relevant) so that you can learn more about the normal physiology of the neonate as well as deviations (Fig. 5.5).

■ Supporting mothers whose babies are on the neonatal unit. If possible, try to spend some time in this unit (see also Chapter 7).

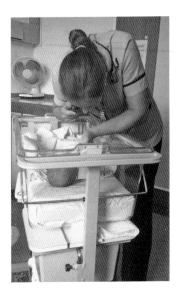

Figure 5.5 Examination of the newborn.

How to prepare

Programmes will vary in the structure of their curricula with respect to high-risk midwifery. Some will focus on the role of the midwife within normality, and there may be limited theoretical content around deviations; likewise, placements may centre on lower risk care. Others will acknowledge that – although the essence of the role of the midwife is in normality – it is inevitable that high-risk situations will be encountered and a greater emphasis may be placed on the theory and practice surrounding this care in collaboration with the wider team. The NMC requires midwives to be proficient in aspects of high-risk care such as referral when deviations from normality occur and management of emergencies. You have previously read extracts from some of the core professional documents in this chapter which also highlight these important aspects of the midwife's role (NMC 2009a, 2012, 2015).

When you have a planned placement

As in all placements, a positive approach and appropriate preparation will best set the scene for your experience. Much of what you have read in other chapters in this book also applies to the context of high-risk placements. Use this guidance to prepare for these allocations, particularly the following:

■ *Read around any available information:* This includes finding out about what the placement has to offer, reading about some of the common complications, conditions or emergencies you may experience, finding out which other professionals and agencies you may encounter as part of the wider interprofessional team.

■ *Visit the placement area and meet some of the staff:* This will help you to alleviate your fears and make you feel that the environment is more familiar when you first start working there. Find out the location of emergency and other key equipment.

■ *Set specific learning objectives:* Focus on the experiences you anticipate gaining in this area which may not have been available in other placements, and how you can relate existing knowledge and skills to this context.

■ *Re-read normal physiology and anatomy:* You will then be better placed to understand the significance of any deviations – as well as to maintain normality as far as possible. For example, understand how hormones interact and the impact these changes can have on body systems such as blood pressure, pulse, renal output and the constituents of blood and urine.

When the unexpected happens

As stated earlier, high-risk situations cannot always be predicted, so preparation may not be possible. It is therefore important that you keep up-to-date with guidelines relating to management of common complications and emergencies so that you can draw on these if an unexpected event occurs (such as in your caseloading practice or when caring for a labouring woman in a midwife-led unit). You also need to familiarise yourself with the environment and location of emergency and other equipment, telephone numbers and on-call rotas (e.g. registrars, consultants and supervisors of midwives) in all clinical areas in which you are placed. Be ready to identify any deviations from normality and refer immediately to your supervising midwife or other relevant professional. Document all observations, care and actions and ensure these are countersigned by the midwife supervising you. In an emergency situation in which you may feel out of your depth watch, listen and participate by scribing and/or supporting the woman – a lot can be learned while you are also fulfilling a vital role in the team. Box 5.1 summarises what you can do to prepare for the unexpected.

Dealing with the fallout

Because of the nature of high-risk midwifery, there is an increased likelihood of follow-up of some sort being required. This may include reporting of incidents (e.g. the use of proformas or Datix). It may also result in a case review or root cause analysis. At times you may be required to write a factual statement of your involvement in a woman's care or your witnessing of others' actions. Try not to be alarmed at the prospect of this, but see it as valuable learning. These activities are not meant to lay blame or be punitive but to provide a means of establishing what happened and whether any changes are needed from an organisational or individual perspective. The purpose is to ensure that safety

and quality of care are maintained for the protection of the public, and that learning is gained about what improvements may be needed for the future. If such a situation arises, it is extremely important that you seek support. This may be from your mentor or the midwife you were working with at the time, a manager or supervisor of midwives or your personal tutor/academic advisor. It is very important that the University is kept informed as they share responsibility for you while you are in placement and need to be able to provide ongoing support and advice. Never write any statements without seeking assistance, as these may be used for institutional, supervisory or staff investigations, by professional bodies or in a court of law.

Midwives (and therefore student midwives) have a professional responsibility to identify or participate in the follow-up of any untoward incidents or issues causing concern. Further information can be found in publications such as 'Midwives Rules and Standards' (NMC 2012) and 'Raising Concerns' (NMC 2013) and 'The Code' (NMC 2015). There is a specific standard relating to this in the latter, which states that we must

> 'Cooperate with all investigations and audits. This includes investigations or audits either against you or relating to others, whether individuals or organisations. It also includes cooperating with requests to act as a witness in any hearing that forms part of an investigation'
>
> (NMC 2015, Standard 23, p 17).

Please find out about your local Trust and University policies with regard to statement writing and escalation of concerns, and seek support from your tutor. Chapter 1 provides further information on this matter.

It is also very important that you have the opportunity to debrief on the experience with an appropriate clinician or member of the academic team. In some situations a group debrief will be arranged; you are encouraged to attend this as you will receive support as well as learning from the experience and how others cope – or not. If you are not given the opportunity for a formal debrief, make sure you speak to someone who can help you come to terms with what happened. It is very useful to talk to someone who was there at the time, such as your mentor or supervising midwife, as they will have knowledge of the details and the actual context in which the experience occurred. However, it can also be helpful to talk to another 'trusted person' – whether clinician or academic. It is also helpful to write a reflection; you may or not wish to include this as part of any formal reflections required in your portfolio or

programme, but the activity of critically analysing an event can lead to increased depth of learning as well as provide you with some closure on the incident.

Conclusion

It is hoped that this chapter has whetted your appetite for being involved in 'high-risk' care, rather than being alarmed by it. To quote Georgia Moffatt, second-year student from Plymouth University:

> 'I find high risk placement is thrilling; I enjoy having to be one step ahead and always thinking. Last year I dreaded epidurals and syntocinon, but since my mentor exposed me to everything constantly it no longer phases me.'

There is so much personal and professional learning to be gained from these experiences. Be reassured that you should be under greater levels of supervision when in this environment, and make best use of the opportunities this provides.

Not only will you learn how to identify and manage conditions and situations, but you will also develop your individual skill set. This will include clinical skills but also those more complex ones such as communication and interpersonal, workload management and prioritisation, decision-making and professional attitudes. You will also grow as a person, discovering new aspects about yourself and your ability to cope with stress and complexity and discovering strategies on how to manage these. You will become more aware of your impact on others and others on you, and your response to this.

You will have a greater understanding of the importance of effective interprofessional teamwork and the essential role communication plays in this. You will have an enhanced appreciation of which other professionals and agencies are available to turn to for advice or to whom to refer women.

Remember that although the role of the midwife is essentially around normality, we have a vital part to play in the care of women for whom things are not straightforward. Learn from and in partnership with them so that you can truly be 'with women' in both low- and high-risk midwifery practice. Even if you don't understand what is going on and others may not have the time to explain, just be there for the women – hold their hand, gently and calmly explain what you can, reassure them that questions you cannot answer will be addressed when the situation has resolved and provide them with comfort and security. It will be hugely satisfying when you can look back and realise that some small action or attitude of yours has made a difference to a woman's experience of her labour, as Georgia demonstrates in her reflection in Vignette 5.5.

Vignette 5.5   Working 'with woman'

'I was caring for a woman in labour who previously had a caesarean section when her cervix was 9 cm dilated. As a student, once it was handed over that this woman's labour was a VBAC, my mind was thinking of the possible risks associated in order to produce a care plan. Once introduced, I was kept busy with observations, CTG analysing, documentation and so on. Her labour was progressing well and she was coping with contractions using the TENS machine. Despite positive information being given, she and her partner would make comments about how "she might as well just go for section". It was at this point that I snapped out of student mode and thought about the woman's psychological well-being. There was no clinical need for a caesarean section, but it was obvious this woman needed a cheerleader – and I was happy to bring out midwifery cheer to increase her confidence in her own abilities, to remind her what she has already achieved and that it was absolutely possible for a vaginal birth. In end the woman had a lovely ventouse birth. The reason why I call it "lovely" is because the registrar and the woman worked together. The choice of words the registrar used made the woman feel empowered. She birthed her own baby!'

Georgia Moffatt
Second-year student, Plymouth University, Devon, UK
Reproduced with permission of Georgia Moffatt.

No voice is more powerful than that of the woman in your care. This chapter draws to a close with the lovely account of a new mother, Laura Woodhouse, explaining how important a student midwife was to her and her husband's experience in Vignette 5.6, and some 'top tips' can be seen in Box 5.2.

Vignette 5.6   A new mother's experience

'My baby was born on 15th of July via caesarean section in the end, as I had reached the point of total exhaustion during the process of induction and [my cervix had] not progressed past 5 cm in 9 hours.

I arrived for my induction already burnt out following a rushed house move two weeks prior to the birth. I'd been burning the candle at both ends in efforts to arrange our new home in a way suited to the arrival of a new baby and this took its toll early during the first afternoon as I drifted off into sleep in one of the hospital cafes! Foolishly, I didn't feel the least bit prepared or adequately rested for the journey of significant physical and emotional strain I was about to embark on. Thank goodness I was fortunate enough to be attended to by some really fantastic people during this difficult time.

I first met the student midwife who ended up being a lifeline for me in the days immediately following the birth late at night after my waters broke. Sara introduced herself and explained her position as a student midwife while she calmly fixed up a monitor, all the while reassuring me with her calm, efficient and quietly competent manner. Very quickly I was in considerable pain and it wasn't long before I had to be moved to a labour room. Once again Sara was there and I couldn't have wished for a nicer person to help me in my time of need as she talked slowly and calmly, always explaining things clearly, giving me the best chance of taking in what she was saying as I dealt with the pain. It's amazing how someone can soothe away some of the fear and anxiety just by speaking but that seemed to be the case with Sara. Whenever I had a question or concern about what was happening, Sara was able to answer in sufficient detail, explaining things of a technical nature in a way that myself and my husband could understand. I know that my husband was particularly grateful that Sara made sure he was fully aware of what was happening as it meant he felt included in the process. This was also true of another student midwife who assisted during the day shift and was present at the birth of my baby boy.

The first night after my son was born Sara was back on shift and I was so pleased to see her when she came to visit in the middle of the night. In the dimly lit ward in the quiet of night we chatted about her studies, and my birth experience. As a mum herself, Sara shared some of her memories of early motherhood and gave me lots of advice, all the while showing genuine empathy, treating me as an individual and not just another person having a baby. When Sara came to visit on the second night post-birth, it was like greeting an old friend, that's how much she'd come to mean

---

to me despite the relatively short space of time. I was touched by Sara's ongoing care for me and my new baby and grateful for her knowledge, experience and patience. Although the pressures of ward shifts must be great, Sara revealed none of this outwardly, something that really impressed me and absolutely what an exhausted and anxious new mum needs. I remain amazed by the genuine care and concern I was shown and I will be forever grateful.'

Laura Woodhouse
New mother (reflecting on the care received from Sara Evans,
third-year student, Plymouth University, Devon, UK)
Reproduced with permission of Laura Woodhouse.

Box 5.2 Top Tips

■ Don't be frightened – embrace the potential learning opportunities.

■ Ensure you are well supported at the time and afterwards.

■ Ask questions (at an appropriate time).

■ Find out about available learning opportunities – talk to fellow students, staff and women in your care; read up information and guidelines.

■ Shadow other health or social care professionals/specialists (e.g. anaesthetists, obstetric and paediatric consultants, perinatal mental health teams, specialist substance misuse midwives, social workers, ultrasonographers, physicians and psychiatrists).

■ Arrange relevant observational visits (e.g. specialist clinics, diagnostic tests and pathology laboratory).

■ Try to follow through the holistic care pathway of women with specific disorders/management – perhaps even during your caseloading (under increased supervision).

■ Read around experiences gained to reinforce learning and help create the links between practice and theory – it will be easier to picture an individual woman than a page of text.

And from fellow Plymouth University students Eloise Fanning, Keri Morter, Mollie Craig and Sophie Denning:

■ Good organisation.

■ Time management.

(continued)

- Communication skills.

- Don't be afraid to ask questions, there is nothing wrong with saying you don't know how to do something.

- Be prepared to get involved and really begin to feel like a member of the interprofessional team.

- In an emergency situation scribe if possible, it's a great way of learning what each member of the team is doing and helps you to find your voice as you have to ask all grades of staff what they are doing, what medications they are giving and so on, and then you can reflect on the documentation alongside the guidelines with your mentor afterwards to develop your understanding.

- If you have time to spare, then making everyone a cup of tea always goes down well.

References

British Association of Perinatal Medicine (2011) Categories of Care 2011. Available at http://www.bapm.org/publications/documents/guidelines/CatsofcarereportAug11.pdf (last accessed 28 July 2014).

International Confederation of Midwives (2008) Position Statement: keeping birth normal. Available at http://internationalmidwives.org/assets/uploads/documents/Position%20Statements%20-%20English/PS2008_007%20ENG%20Keeping%20Birth%20Normal.pdf (last accessed 28 July 2014).

Mothers and Babies: Reducing Risk through Audits and Confidential Enquiries across the UK (MBRRACE-UK) (2014) Saving lives, improving mothers' care. National Perinatal Epidemiology Unit, Oxford. Available at https://www.npeu.ox.ac.uk/downloads/files/mbrrace-uk/reports/Saving%20Lives%20Improving%20Mothers%20Care%20report%202014%20Full.pdf (last accessed 24 February 2015).

McCandlish R, Bowler U, van Asten, H, et al. (1998) A randomized controlled trial of care of the perineum during the second stage of normal labour. Br J Obstet Gynaecol 105: 1262–1272.

National Institute for Health and Care Excellence (2011) Antenatal care pathway. Available at http://pathways.nice.org.uk/pathways/antenatal-care (last accessed 28 July 2014).

Nicholls L, Webb C (2006) What makes a good midwife? An integrative review of methodologically-diverse research. J Adv Nurs 56 (4): 414–429.

Nursing and Midwifery Council (2007) Standards for medicines management. Nursing and Midwifery Council, London. Available at http://www.nmc-uk.org/Documents/NMC-Publications/NMC-Standards-for-medicines-management.pdf (last accessed 28 July 2014).

Nursing and Midwifery Council (2009a) Standards for pre-registration midwifery education. Nursing and Midwifery Council, London. Available at http://www.nmc-uk.org/Documents/NMC-Publications/nmc

StandardsforPre_RegistrationMidwifery Education.pdf (last accessed 28 July 2014).

Nursing and Midwifery Council (2009b) Record keeping: guidance for nurses and midwives. Nursing and Midwifery Council, London. Available at http://www.nmc-uk .org/Documents/NMC-Publications/NMC-Record-Keeping-Guidance.pdf (last accessed 28 July 2014).

Nursing and Midwifery Council (2012) Midwives Rules and Standards 2012. Nursing and Midwifery Council, London. Available at http://www.nmc-uk.org/Documents/NMC-Publications/Midwives%20Rules%20and%20Standards%20(Plain)%20FINAL.pdf (last accessed 28 July 2014).

Nursing and Midwifery Council (2013) Raising concerns: guidance for nurses and midwives. Nursing and Midwifery Council, London. Available at http://wwwnrdrr.nmc-ukrrdrr.org/Documents/NMC-Publications/NMC-Raising-and-escalating-concernsrrdrr .pdf (last accessed 28 July 2014).

Nursing and Midwifery Council (2015) The Code: professional standards of practice and behaviour for nurses and midwives. Nursing and Midwifery Council, London. Available at http://www.nmc-uk.org/The-revised-Code/ (last accessed 24 February 2015).

Skirton H, Stephen N, Doris F, Cooper M, Avis M, Fraser DM (2012) Preparedness of newly qualified midwives to deliver care: an evaluation of pre-registration midwifery education through an analysis of key events. *Midwifery* 28 (5): e660–e666. Available at http://www.midwiferyjournal.com/article/S0266-6138(11)00121-5/abstract (last accessed 28 July 2014).

Winter C, Crofts J, Laxton C, Bamfield S, Draycott T (eds) (2012) *Practical Obstetric Multi-Professional Training Course Manual*, 2nd edition. RCOG Press, London.

Further resources

International Confederation of Midwives: www .internationalmidwives.org.

National Institute for Health and Care Excellence: www.nice.org.uk.

Nursing and Midwifery Council: www.nmc-uk .org.

Perinatal Institute: www.perinatal.org.uk.

Royal College of Midwives: www.rcm.org.uk.

Royal College of Obstetricians and Gynaecologists: www.rcog.org.uk.

The Cochrane Library: www.thecochranelibrary .com.

Chapter 6
CASELOADING

Stella Rawnson

Introduction

Caseloading practice can be a really exciting and enjoyable part of your midwifery education. It gives you an opportunity to build meaningful relationships with women and develop confidence and competence in essential skills for midwifery practice. Careful planning and preparation will enable you to gain the most from this experience and lessen any anxieties you may have. This chapter provides lots of hints and tips to help you in this. Any persons referred to in this chapter have had their names and identities changed so as to protect confidentiality (NMC 2015 newly published standards).

Back to the beginning

Often new ideas and suggestions for how learning can be improved come from students and this was how the idea of including caseloading practice as part of midwifery education first came about. Student midwife caseload holding was first introduced at Bournemouth University (BU) in 1996

by two enthusiastic and forward-thinking student midwives and their midwifery lecturers. The students suggested the idea, because they felt they could only 'dip in and out' of women's care during pregnancy and childbirth, mainly because clinical practice time was split between many short placements in different maternity care settings. So, caseloading practice was developed in order to give students an experience of providing continuity of care to women throughout their pregnancies and into the postnatal period (Lewis et al. 2008). Bournemouth University made a decision to include student caseloading practice within midwifery education for all students in 2001 (Rawnson et al. 2008). This raised much interest in the United Kingdom and abroad. As a result, many universities all over the world now include caseloading as part of their midwifery educational programmes (Aune et al. 2011; Gray et al. 2013).

New standards were set in 2009 by the Nursing and Midwifery Council (NMC) which stated that student midwives must have an opportunity to experience continuity of care through caseload practice. So, if you are studying midwifery in the United

The Hands-on Guide to Midwifery Placements, First Edition.
Edited by Luisa Cescutti-Butler and Margaret Fisher.
© 2016 John Wiley & Sons, Ltd. Published 2016 by John Wiley & Sons, Ltd.

Kingdom, it will form a compulsory aspect of the practice-based element of your educational programme. As well as exposing students to new ways of working, this change in educational strategy reflects the move towards woman-centred care within the NHS in recent years

What is student midwife caseloading practice?

The aim of midwifery education programmes is to develop competent midwives who are ready to provide care for women in the real world of midwifery practice. Caseloading practice is seen as a learning experience that enables students to move towards achieving this goal by developing their knowledge, skills and confidence in supporting women in normal childbirth. Carrying a personal caseload enables students to work in a more independent way (with support from their supervising mentor) and be actively involved in clinical decision-making and care planning for the women in their caseload. When you have a student caseload under the supervision of your midwife mentor you will provide care and support to a group of women throughout their pregnancy, labour, birth and the early days of parenting, until midwifery care is completed (NMC 2009).

Student caseloading is designed to enable you to

■ understand the impact of pregnancy, birth and the addition of a new baby(ies) to a woman and her family's life;

■ learn about the practicalities of organising, planning and providing woman-centred midwifery care;

■ understand the importance of and develop skills in leadership, self-management, problem-solving and clinical decision-making; and

■ have an opportunity to work in a more independent way, while under the supervision and support of your midwife mentor.

Organisation of learning experience

How you will experience caseload practice varies across universities. Depending on your University you may begin caseloading during the first year and continue throughout your programme, do it in the second and third years or undertake it in your final year.

The number of women you provide care for during this experience also varies across universities. In Australia for example, students in some universities are expected to provide continuity of care for up to 30 women (Rolls & McGuinness 2007; Gray et al. 2013; Browne & Taylor 2014). In the standards set by the Nursing and Midwifery Council for UK midwifery education, it is clearly stated that students will care for a 'group of women' during caseloading practice (NMC 2009). This means students are expected to commit to undertake care for a number of women. Taking on a group of women rather than just one, provides the opportunity for a truly meaningful learning experience.

It is most likely that during caseload practice you will build a personal caseload of women. What is meant by a personal caseload and how students choose women to caseload also varies across universities. Your personal caseload of women may for example be made up of either a fixed number of women or a number you have personally negotiated. The women may have been assigned to you, or you and your mentor might have invited them to be part of your caseload. They may be women who are already part of your mentor's caseload for whom you undertake the planning and provision of care.

Advantages of caseloading practice

Before you take on your caseload, it is worth considering how you as a student

midwife might personally benefit from caseloading practice as well as how receiving care from you throughout her entire childbearing journey might impact on a woman's pregnancy and birth experience. Reflect on Ania's situation (Box 6.2) and how you might benefit from caseloading her.

Working with Ania might help you develop a range of skills including accessing local Polish support groups. It may also enhance your confidence in communicating with and caring for women. Ania may benefit enormously from the extra input you can offer her as part of your caseload.

Box 6.2   Ania

Ania is Polish and has recently moved from Poland to your local area to join her husband who is a chef in a restaurant in a nearby town. She is 14 weeks pregnant with her first child and has agreed to be part of your caseload. Ania and her husband are very excited about the pregnancy but know very little about maternity care services or birthing options. They both have a good grasp of English and have learnt to speak it fairly fluently.

Students' views and experiences

When students were interviewed for research carried out in the United Kingdom, Australia and Norway (Rawnson et al. 2009; Aune et al. 2011; Rawnson 2011; Gray et al. 2013) this is what they felt about caseloading (Fig. 6.1):

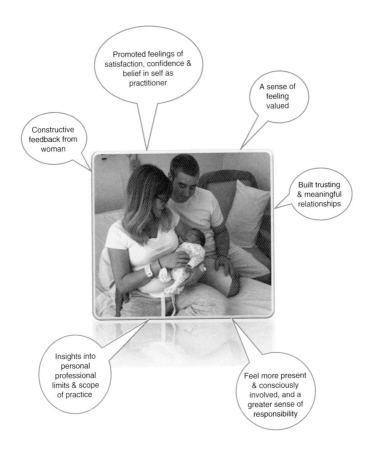

Promoted feelings of satisfaction, confidence & belief in self as practitioner

A sense of feeling valued

Constructive feedback from woman

Built trusting & meaningful relationships

Insights into personal professional limits & scope of practice

Feel more present & consciously involved, and a greater sense of responsibility

Figure 6.1 Perceived benefits.

A sense of feeling valued

■ Students felt they got to know the individual women within their caseload and built meaningful relationships with them and their families. This is because they felt they got to know the women on a more personal level, gaining an understanding of their anxieties, hopes and dreams for their pregnancy.

■ They felt welcomed as care providers, and trusted and valued as knowledgeable practitioners. Being valued in this way appeared to strengthen students' commitment to the women in their caseload.

■ Establishing these close relationships and feeling valued by the women promoted a sense of satisfaction amongst students, which contributed to their enjoyment of caseloading practice.

Working more independently

■ Students are always supervised by a midwife mentor during clinical practice. During caseloading, rather than close shadowing this supervision was often reported as being indirect, where students provided care on their own without their mentor present.

■ Working in this way stimulated a strong sense of responsibility amongst students to ensure high-quality care provision. Many reported undertaking additional study to research topics to ensure the information they gave in response to the women's questions was evidenced-based. Students also talked about their desire to act as advocates for the women within their care by supporting and championing their birthing choices.

■ Having this greater independence and freedom to practise in their own way opened students' eyes to what it will be like to practise as a qualified midwife. It prompted them to reflect on where they were, in terms of their clinical skill development and knowledge base.

Belief in self as practitioner

■ Students reported being more actively involved and taking greater responsibility in clinical decision-making and care planning for the women within their caseload. This often required them to liaise and work more closely with other health care providers.

■ Students felt that because they provided care to each of the women within their caseload throughout their entire childbearing journey, their learning and clinical skills had grown in all areas. They reported a newfound confidence and belief in their clinical competence.

■ Receiving constructive feedback from the women within their caseload on the care they had organised and provided was also important to students. Many reported how the woman's appreciative comments boosted and reinforced their confidence and sense of belief in themselves as a practitioner.

Organisational and leadership skills

■ In working to achieve quality care provision for the women in their caseload, students reported they had become more skilful in self-leadership. Many talked about gaining insight into aspects of their practice that needed further development and working to achieve this.

■ Students also reported that through working flexibly to provide holistic woman-centred care for the various women within their caseload they had greatly developed their time management and organisational skills.

Students seem to agree caseloading practice is an enormously enjoyable and satisfying experience. For some students, it not only boosted their confidence and knowledge but also changed their ideas about how they wanted to work once qualified as a midwife. Like one of the student midwives who first initiated student caseloading at Bournemouth University, they wanted to go directly into a caseloading scheme (Rawnson 2011). While some opportunities exist within contemporary practice to work in this way, midwife caseload-holding in its purest form in the United Kingdom really sits in domains outside the NHS such as Independent Midwifery group practice.

However, managing the day-to-day practicalities of carrying a personal caseload alongside home and University academic commitments is not without its challenges!

As you will read elsewhere in this book, reflective writing is encouraged in midwifery. This reflection has been written to illustrate some of the challenges and rewards you may come across as a student midwife taking on a caseload (Fig. 6.2). Like the students in the studies, we have looked at these tend to be around balancing the competing pressures of flexible working, being on-call

and being available to attend women in labour at short notice. Similar to Jo, students also talked about a strong sense of responsibility to ensure high-quality care provision for the women within their caseload, and a fear of letting women down.

Jo Lake shares her reflection on carrying a personal caseload in Vignette 6.1.

Reflecting on personal priorities for care

Before considering the practicalities of how to plan and provide care for women during caseloading, it can help to first put ourselves under the microscope. In life, we often have many different roles, for example, being a sister/brother, mother/father, partner/lover, girl/boyfriend and student/employee. These roles inform the way in which we act and perform tasks in terms of what we consider to be appropriate behaviour.

It's almost as if we have a series of 'hats' that we put on and take off throughout the day as we move in and out of our different roles. We act differently depending on which 'hat' we are wearing. Yet inside we are the same person. So, while we may conduct ourselves differently depending on which 'hat' we put on, the way in which we behave in that role will be influenced by our personality, personal beliefs and values (Fig. 6.3).

Once you start your midwifery training the role of 'student midwife' is another 'hat' that you will wear. I

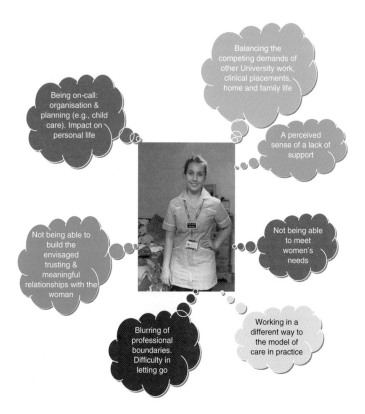

Figure 6.2 Perceived challenges.

therefore urge you to think honestly about your beliefs, values and priorities around how you will provide woman-centred care. This is because every action you take in caring for the women in your caseload will be influenced by your personal knowledge and under-standing of what is important in life; your 'personal philosophy'. The impor-tance of this during caseloading practice is illustrated in Heather's story below. Heather was a student who participated in my research (Rawnson 2011). Using her own words, she describes her dilemma and what she learned from it.

> 'Skin-to-skin is a particular little bug bear of mine I suppose, a hobby horse. Although I desperately wanted all my ladies to have skin-to-skin in fact one of them didn't, one of them chose not to. And I found that I

Vignette 6.1   Reflection on carrying a personal caseload

During the second year of my Midwifery degree, I took on a caseload of five pregnant women who were of low- and high-risk status as I felt that this would be of most benefit to me, enabling me not only to get to grips with some complex pregnancy-related conditions but also to nurture personal intuition and vital skills for promoting normality in every woman's pregnancy, childbirth or postnatal experience. Each of the women on my caseload had due dates at different times which meant I was consistently kept busy for a period of about a year.

I cannot say that caseloading has been easy. At each appointment, you can be presented with something out of the ordinary, such as a high blood pressure, excessive weight loss in the newborn or reduced fetal movements, and you realise that you are responsible for initiating an appropriate plan of care. Of course, your supervising midwife is often only at the end of the telephone but in that moment the woman is looking to you for advice and reassurance. In these situations, the question 'What should I do now?' goes through your mind dozens of time as you carry out your clinical assessment, weighing up the severity of the risk that is posed and ultimately choosing an appropriate path for the woman and her unborn baby.

I am also conscious that due to my personal nature I have remained apprehensive about so many of the small details throughout my caseloading experience; worrying myself over different bits of paperwork or wondering if I would even hear my telephone ringing at night-time. However, with each woman I've cared for there have been numerous occasions when I've felt at ease, peaceful even. These moments were usually when I was sat on the sofa side by side with the woman I was caring for, answering questions and offering reassurance and encouragement. Or when I quietly slipped out of the labour room leaving mum, dad and baby in one another's arms, content and restful. And it is during these times that I begun to realise how precious the student–mother relationship is.

Following personal reflection and discussion with my peers I have come to the conclusion that student caseloading can have a positive effect on many aspects of the woman's pregnancy and childbirth journey, including the type of delivery she has, her infant feeding choices or even a reduction in her level of anxiety around the reality of having a baby. I believe it's no coincidence that four out of the five women on my caseload had normal vaginal births (the last woman had an elective caesarean at 36 weeks gestation due to an underlying medical condition which prevented her from allowing herself to go into labour naturally), using minimal pain relief, and all five were breastfeeding when I discharged them at 3–4 weeks postnatal.

In addition to this, I have received some verbal feedback from the women I've been caseloading that has impacted and encouraged me more than they'll ever know. The first woman I caseloaded told me that she would have been really scared if I hadn't been there for her labour and birth. How wonderful to think that as student midwives we can play a key part in breaking the vicious cycle of fear that can negatively impact on a woman's birthing process, leading to a

(*continued*)

cascade of interventions that result in an abundance of more fear! Another of my caseloading women said to me "I've realised that I have a choice in relation to everything surrounding my pregnancy and birth." Again, this was a light-bulb moment for me. If only every woman was granted with such enlightenment and empowerment from their care providers, I wonder if their experiences of pregnancy and birth might be completely different.

Caseloading is also very important for building a student midwife's confidence. Too often, students can feel like a third wheel in the antenatal clinic or on the labour ward. I've had some experiences, particularly early on in my training where I've felt as though I could quietly slip out of the room and no one would even notice. However, the order of things is turned on its head when you begin to manage your own caseload of women. In the labour room, the woman is looking to you for support and guidance, she wants to ask your advice regarding what pain relief is available, and she even wants to photograph you with her baby when it's all over! She will never forget you!

There is no denying that trying to fit placement, University assessments and some form of family/social life around caseloading is extremely difficult and yet another lesson in the unpredictability of childbirth. I remember my University tutors really emphasising being on call as the most demanding aspect of caseloading. However, in my experience the most challenging part has been coordinating the women's postnatal visits alongside placement or University lectures. Since babies will arrive when they are ready it is impossible to predict when you will be going out to do visits after the birth. Being flexible during the antenatal period is much more easily accomplished where I was able to book in my visits at times that suited everyone. But postnatally I often found I was rushing round to do postnatal checks at 5 p.m. due to other commitments. On these occasions, I hoped that the woman hadn't felt abandoned all day and that the midwife accompanying me (or on the other end of the phone if I was visiting unaccompanied) wasn't frustrated by me undertaking a visit so late in the day. I desperately wanted to give the woman the time and attention she deserved as a new mother and yet as a student midwife I was being pulled in so many different directions.

My heart tells me that caseloading is totally worth all the anxiety, stress and on-calls. As student midwives, we are in a privileged position where we witness a woman flourishing throughout her pregnancy journey, birth experience and postnatal expedition. Not only do we witness it but we can positively influence it. Not everything will be 'normal' within a woman's childbearing experience but we can do so much to provide 'normality' to the women under our care. I personally have been able to support a woman who had a history of postnatal depression but expressed how she enjoyed the postnatal period with her new son far more this time because she felt so well supported. I also supported a woman through an elective caesarean and enjoyed the challenge of making this experience as natural and enjoyable as it could possibly be. And sometimes just a familiar face can make all the difference to a woman who is experiencing anxiety or trepidation regarding childbirth's unknowns.

I believe caseloading is an experience that simultaneously manages to stretch and refine each student midwife in a unique way. It prepares a student midwife for autonomous practice, pushing them to their limits in relation to prioritisation, time-management and decision-making. The process encourages students to give of themselves to the women under their care; a philosophy that can quickly dwindle when newly qualified midwives are thrown into the reality of a busy labour-ward environment. I believe you get out of caseloading what you put in. The greater the commitment to the women you are caring for, the more rewards you will reap in return. As a supernumerary member of my community team, I chose not to feel guilty about attending 1-hour long antenatal appointments or 2-hour long post-natal checks with the women on my caseload, because I know that this is the gold standard, the care that they need and appreciate. I also know that in the long run spending time with woman will teach me greater intuition than a textbook ever could.

I extend my gratitude to the women who entrusted themselves and their babies into my care and my midwifery mentors who supported me throughout the process enabling me to grow, learn and adapt in my role as a midwife-to-be.

Jo Lake
Third-year student, Bournemouth University, Dorset, UK
Reproduced with permission of Jo Lake

had to really examine how I communicated with her once she'd let me know that she didn't want it. She wanted the baby taken away [at birth] and dried and wrapped up [before she cuddled him/ her] . . . I knew obviously that I had to support her, but it was quite difficult for me to get over my own prejudices I suppose in that instance, and I hope I did'.

Practicalities of planning and providing care (living the reality)

In this section, we discuss the 'nitty-gritty' of caseloading practice; the 'what' and 'how' of organising and managing your personal caseload. Set out below are the aspects of caseloading practice that are likely to be common to most University programmes, with insights to help you to decide what will work best for you.

Building a personal caseload

As Jo reflected in Vignette 6.1 carrying a personal caseload, while a fantastic learning experience, can prove challenging at times. It is therefore important students build realistic caseloads that 'fit' their individual personal circumstances (Fry et al. 2008).

Size of caseload

■ If you could choose, how many women would you like to caseload? In thinking about this, remember that you cannot let women down or raise false expectations. If you invite a woman to be part of your caseload, you cannot at a

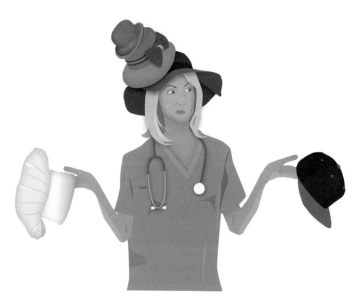

Figure 6.3 HATS. Reproduced with permission of Hugo Beaumont.

later date decide that you no longer wish to provide care for her unless exceptional circumstances exist.

■ Think about your personal life, do you have family, childcare or other commitments that need to be taken into consideration? Will these commitments limit the number of women that you can realistically care for?

■ Are you someone who struggles with academic assignment deadlines? Is this an aspect of the midwifery programme that you think you will need to invest a lot of extra time over and above that suggested by the University? How will you maintain your caseload alongside this commitment?

■ Some students find the best way to work out what size of caseload is best for them is to initially recruit one or two women to their caseload, then gradually add more women as their caseloading experience progresses.

Transport

■ Are you a car driver? Do you have 24-hour access to your own independent transport such as a car, motorbike or scooter? Remember, public transport in your practice placement area may not be provided or be of limited availability at night, bank holidays and weekends.

■ Not having 24-hour access to your own car, motorbike or scooter may therefore limit your choices in terms of inviting women to be part of your caseload, for example you may need to recruit women choosing hospital birth rather than home birth.

Timescale

■ If you could choose, when would be the best time for the women in your caseload to give birth? In thinking about this, it is important to remember that a normal pregnancy can last between 37 and 42 weeks.

■ How will you cope with being on-call in order to attend women during labour and birth? Are you someone who would prefer to get it over in one hit and be on-call for one block period of time or would you prefer to have spaced-out, shorter periods of on-call? Remember, you could be on-call for a period of up to 5 weeks for each woman.

■ Do you have important events – for example elective placements, family holidays and assignment deadlines that you need to think about when planning?

■ Your caseloading experience won't end until the woman's postnatal midwifery care is completed and has been handed over to the health visitor. When planning your caseloading timescale, it may therefore be useful to work backwards, that is, from when care provision needs to be completed.

Inviting women to be part of your caseload

■ Women should never feel 'pressured' to agree to be part of your caseload.

How will you make sure they have a genuine choice?

■ At Bournemouth University, students often discuss caseloading with the woman at the initial midwife's 'booking consultation' appointment but do not invite her to be part of their caseload. The student's midwife mentor will contact the woman at a later date for this purpose. This is because women often find it hard to say 'no' in a face-to-face conversation with the student.

■ So that they can make an informed choice, it is important that women understand exactly what they are being asked to agree to, in other words what being part of a student's caseload will mean for them. Some universities provide a letter for women containing this information, others may ask students to design and develop their own leaflet for this purpose.

■ Before you invite women to be part of your caseload, think carefully about what level of commitment you can offer and be prepared to commit to deliver on it. This may involve getting agreement and support from your family or the people you live with.

Communication pathways

The secret to successful caseload-holding is keeping everyone involved fully informed of what you are doing – the women, midwives, University and so on. Communication pathways between yourself, your mentor and the women in your care, should be discussed and agreed before you begin caseloading practice (Fry et al. 2011). This is because you may at times, as Jo described, work independently without direct supervision from your mentor.

Here are some communication issues to consider:

■ How will the women in your care contact you to arrange appointments, discuss health queries or let you know they have gone into labour? Remember, social media networking sites, for example, Facebook cannot be used for this purpose.

■ How will you contact your mentor or other members of the team to discuss the care you have given and/or any questions or concerns you may have?

■ Will your local NHS Trust or University provide you with a pager or mobile phone, or will you be expected to organise your own communication method?

■ Some students choose to use their personal mobile phone. This can work well but it does mean that when caseloading care is ended the woman will still have your contact number. Using a separate phone for caseloading practice may therefore be something to think about.

At the beginning of the caseloading relationship, it helps to set 'ground rules' so that each woman who agrees to be part of your personal caseload clearly understands what your role is and what you can and can't offer.

Consider Amy's case study below Box 6.3.

Amy's case study shows the importance of explaining your role clearly to women so misunderstandings don't arise. It also highlights why effective communication pathways and professional support networks are essential during caseloading practice.

These guidelines will help you develop effective ground rules for caseloading practice:

■ Students should not be the first point of contact in an emergency or where urgent care is required. The information provided to women should clearly signpost the contact numbers to call in these situations, so appropriate care can be accessed.

Box 6.3   Amy

Amy is pregnant with her second child. She moved to the area recently and doesn't have family or friends living locally. Her husband is a lorry driver and is often away for long periods of time, leaving Amy to care for their 3-year-old son Zak. You have started to receive texts and phone calls from Amy often quite late, around 8 or 9 p.m., when Zak is asleep. Mostly these have been questions about keeping healthy during pregnancy but once Amy raised a concern about her baby's well-being. You are worried that if you don't respond to her calls or texts that you might miss something vital and Amy and/or her baby's health will suffer.

■ Women should always have direct access to a qualified midwife. Contact numbers should be given so that women can speak to a midwife without having to go through their caseloading student first.

■ It is useful to identify times during the working day when women can contact you to arrange appointments or discuss non-urgent health questions, for example, 9 a.m.–5 p.m., Monday to Friday. For ground rules to be effective it is important to work within the timeframe agreed. If, as in Amy's case study, you respond to texts or phone calls outside of the timescale set, women will think that it's acceptable to contact you at these times.

■ Women should understand that while you will be on-call for them during their labour and birth, when the time comes you may not be able to attend. You cannot absolutely promise to be at the birth as issues beyond your control may arise that prevent you such as personal illness, car breakdown or you could be on shift and caring for another labouring woman.

Role and responsibilities

Once enrolled as a midwifery student, you have a responsibility to behave professionally. You must be open and honest, act with integrity and maintain the reputation of the midwifery profession at all times (NMC 2015). To ensure the safety and well-being of the women within your care during caseloading practice, it's essential that this responsibility is recognised and upheld. This is vital,

because women will place their trust in you. The following pointers offer guidance on how to work as a safe and effective practitioner:

Maintaining professional relationships

With your mentor(s)

■ Remember that at all times, even when you provide care without your mentor present, your mentor is fully responsible for the midwifery care the women in your caseload receive. This responsibility includes all of your actions, including any mistakes you make.

■ This means that mentors must monitor the care you give to check that they are satisfied with what you have done. If at any time they have concerns about the quality of care you are providing, they must intervene. Your mentor will discuss this with you and correct any errors or omissions.

■ Caseloading practice can provide opportunities to work more independently. You might, for example, visit a woman at home on your own to provide care, reporting back to your mentor afterwards. Working like this can really boost your confidence and professional development. However, your mentor won't agree to this unless they are confident in your ability to perform to the required standard when they are not directly with you.

■ It may help to spend some time working with your mentor before you begin caseloading practice, so your mentor can assess your level of knowledge and competence.

With women

- Close bonds are often formed as students' journey with women through pregnancy, birth and the early days of parenting. Building these meaningful relationships with women is often an enjoyable part of caseloading practice.

- It is important however, that professional boundaries are maintained within the caseloading relationship. Students need to distinguish the fine line between being a professional friend and a personal friend.

- These close relationships can encourage a strong sense of responsibility and commitment in students. However, remember that you are not a 24-hour help-line or counselling service.

- Your mentor will need to intervene if it seems you may be having difficulty in maintaining appropriate boundaries.

Safe and effective practitioner

Being a safe and effective practitioner requires you to think about your clinical competence, confidence and knowledge. What can you do well, and what areas do you need to develop? Talk to your mentor(s) about this so they can support you appropriately.

- Remember that risk status during pregnancy can change and women can develop complications. If this happens, you will need increased support and your mentor may need to play a more active role in care delivery.

- At no point during caseloading practice should a student feel out of their depth. If at any time, you are unsure how to provide care to women in your caseload you must seek immediate guidance and support from your mentor and/or supervisor of midwives.

- Your safety matters. When visiting women at home on your own you must always follow your local NHS Trust 'Lone working policy'.

- When thinking about keeping yourself safe and well, be aware that caseloading practice can be emotionally challenging at times. Take time out to reflect on your feelings and access appropriate support when you need it. Talk to your mentor, supervisor of midwives, friends and family about your concerns, although you need of course to consider confidentiality issues.

- Students should work not more than 48 hours per week. It is therefore a good idea to keep a record of all the caseloading clinical hours you work and discuss with your mentor when you can take 'time back' if necessary.

- Despite what is sometimes shown on television, some labours go on for a long time! Negotiating with your mentor to take regular rest breaks may therefore be appropriate. Eat regularly and keep yourself hydrated.

Record keeping

- Accurate record keeping is a significant part of caseloading practice. You must keep a record of all contacts you have with each woman, for example phone calls and texts. This record should include the date and time of contact, the advice given and any action taken.

- It is also a good idea to keep track of when you last saw each woman and when their next appointment is scheduled.

- Full and accurate records of the care you provide should be documented in the woman's hand-held maternity notes and/or hospital notes, as appropriate.

- The records that you keep should be checked and countersigned by your mentor. When midwifery care is completed, these records will be filed in the woman's maternity notes.

Women's views and experiences

As well as students reporting many advantages of caseloading practice, pregnant women also feel they benefit from being cared for in this way. Knowing how positively women view it should fuel your enthusiasm for caseloading practice.

Only a few small studies have looked at women's experiences of receiving continuity of care from a student midwife. However, much work has been done exploring women's experiences of care provision from qualified midwives through schemes enabling continuity of carer. These studies show women really value being cared for through such schemes. Women felt they built trusting relationships with their midwife, had a greater sense of control over their birthing experiences, and were more confident and highly satisfied with the care they received (McCourt et al. 1998; Homer et al. 2002; Sandall et al.

2013). Links between caseload midwifery and positive birth outcomes have also been demonstrated. These include less risk of birth interventions, a higher number of natural births and less use of epidurals (Sandall et al. 2013). Some studies have also shown a reduced risk of caesarean birth (McCourt et al. 1998; Benjamin et al. 2001). While this evidence relates to midwives who caseload, it is possible that such positive outcomes could equally have parallels with students who caseload.

For my doctorate, I am conducting a research study to find out what women think and feel about being part of a student midwife's caseload (Rawnson 2014). I hope to paint a picture here of what it meant to the women who participated in my research as well as in studies conducted in Australia and Norway to receive care from a student throughout their entire childbearing journey (Rolls & McGuinness 2007; Aune et al. 2012; Browne & Taylor 2014).

Wanting to contribute to student learning

Women really wanted to help their student learn and felt that by agreeing to be part of their caseload, they could contribute to the student's education.

'The thing for me is everybody needs to learn and you've got to start somewhere and if people like myself don't give people the opportunity to do their studies, then how are they going to get their experience or knowledge?' (Jody*, 34 years old and gave birth to her second child) (* Not her real name).

Valuing continuity of carer

Women identified continuity of student care throughout their childbearing experience as being very important, and suggested this was something that other mothers would benefit from having.

'I'm really edgy this time but I think having Carla [student] makes it better, makes me feel a bit better about it all 'cause I think at least there's someone else there along the journey' (Kelly*, 25 years old and pregnant with her fourth baby).

Like the women who were cared for through midwifery continuity of carer schemes, the women in my study felt they built strong bonds and a trusting relationship with their student. They felt the student understood them, and the care they wanted during labour. Because they felt that the student was close to them as individuals, they found the student's presence during care reassuring.

'It's nice if she [student] can make it to the birth, it'd be like having almost like a friend who you've built up a relationship with there, like having your mate there almost' (Kelly).

Enhanced care

Women felt their student was genuinely interested in them and cared about them.

'She's [student] really excited as well which is really nice because it's just making it a little bit more personal. I'm not just some lady who's having a baby I'm Anna, I'm actually her first case as well so I know I'll be a bit special to her and she'll be special to me as well because it's my first

baby' (Anna*, 38 years old and pregnant with her first baby).

They felt they could Trust in the student's ability to care for them, and that they were in safe hands. The student would know how best to advise or support them, they only had to call.

'She's [student] been brilliant when I've seen her and she's really cheery and friendly and it's, it's just like having a midwife. I don't realise the difference, she asks the same questions, does the same things it's just the same as having a midwife, really. I Trust her; she's a midwife to me' (Kelly).

This enabled them to feel more empowered during their childbearing and early parenting experiences, promoting feelings of satisfaction with their care experiences (Fig. 6.4).

'At the hospital [for the birth] it was like when she [student] turned up it was, like that's it, familiar face! I know, I know you are going to help me, I know that you know what my fears are. When she turned up I said 'right that's it Pippa's here, she's gonna sort me out, she's gonna look after me' and that was good because I knew that she wouldn't let anything happen to me' (Jody).

Conclusion

This chapter has outlined what caseloading practice is and how you can prepare yourself for undertaking it. To help you think about this, it has highlighted the benefits for women and for students and incorporated helpful hints and tips to help you manage some of the perceived

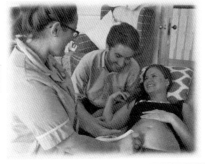

Developed trusting & therapeutic relationships

Continuity was important for women & their partners

Care highly rated

Promoted feelings of satisfaction

Presence and offers of physical & emotional support appreciated

Felt more empowered during childbearing & early parenting experiences

Figure 6.4 Women's experiences.

Box 6.4 Top Tips

■ Keep to the hours that you agree to be available for non-urgent calls.

■ Order a free SIM card and put in an old phone. This provides a dedicated 'hotline' for your caseloading women that can be switched off out of agreed hours.

■ Think carefully about the on-call commitment and how it will fit alongside your home and University work.

■ Pack yourself a 'birth bag'. Include things you will need when going to a birth for example uniform, work shoes, food, and drink. Make sure everyone you live with knows where it is kept in case they need to bring it to you.

■ If you are restricted to public transport, set aside a taxi fund in case you need to get to a home birth, birth centre or hospital out of hours.

■ Always let your mentors know that you are on-call, so that they understand if you have to leave mid-shift, arrive late or unable to work a shift.

Students from Bournemouth University, Dorset, UK

challenges you may come across. Student reflective accounts included in the chapter illustrate the learning you can gain from caseloading for midwifery practice. They also reveal how rewarding and enjoyable it can be to truly provide one-to-one care for women who choose to become part of your caseload.

References

Aune I, Dahlberg U, Ingbrigtsen O (2011) Relational care as a model of care in practical midwifery studies. *Br J Midwifery* 19: 515–523.

Aune I, Dahlberg U, Ingbrigtsen O (2012) Parents' experiences of midwifery students providing continuity of care. *Midwifery* 28: 432–438.

Benjamin Y, Walsh D, Toub N (2001) A comparison of partnership caseload midwifery care with conventional team midwifery care: labour and birth outcomes. *Midwifery* 17: 234–240.

Browne J, Taylor J (2014) 'It's a good thing . . . ': women's views on their continuity experiences with midwifery students from one Australian region. *Midwifery* 30: e108–e114.

Fry J, Rawnson S, Lewis P (2008) Student midwife caseloading – preparing and supporting students. *Br J Midwifery* 16: 568–595.

Fry J, Rawnson S, Lewis P (2011) Problems and Practicalities in student caseload holding. *Br J Midwifery* 19: 659–666.

Gray J, Leap N, Sheehy A, Homer SE (2013) Students' perceptions of the follow-through experience in 3 year bachelor of midwifery programmes in Australia. *Midwifery* 29: 400–406.

Homer CS, Davis GK, Cooke M, Barclay LM (2002) Women's experiences of continuity of midwifery care in a randomised controlled trial in Australia. *Midwifery* 18: 102–112.

Lewis P, Fry J, Rawnson S (2008) Student midwife caseloading – a new approach to midwifery education. *Br J Midwifery* 16: 499–502.

New standards published (2015) *The Code: Standards of Conduct, Performance and Ethics for Nurses and Midwives.* NMC, London.

Nursing and Midwifery Council [NMC] (2009) *Standards for pre-registration midwifery education.* NMC, London.

Nursing and Midwifery Council [NMC] (2015) *Guidance on professional conduct for nursing and midwifery students.* NMC, London.

McCourt C, Page L, Hewison J, Vail A (1998) Evaluation of one-to-one midwifery: women's responses to care. *Birth* 25: 73–80.

Rawnson S (2011) A qualitative study exploring student midwives experiences of carrying a caseload as part of their midwifery education in England. *Midwifery* 27: 786–792.

Rawnson S (2014) Listening to women: exploring women's experiences of being part of a student midwife's caseload. PhD thesis. Bournemouth University. (unpublished).

Rawnson S, Brown S, Wilkins C, Leamon J (2009) Student midwives' views of caseloading: the BUMP study. *Br J Midwifery* 17: 484–489.

Rawnson S, Fry J, Lewis P (2008) Student caseloading: embedding the concept within education. *Br J Midwifery* 16: 636–641.

Rolls C, McGuinness B (2007) Women's experiences of a Follow Through Journey Program with Bachelor of Midwifery students. *Women Birth* 20: 149–152.

Sandall J, Soltani H, Gates S, Shennan A, Devane D (2013) Midwife-led continuity models versus other models of care for childbearing women. *Cochrane Database Syst Rev* Issue 8. Art. No.: CD004667. DOI: 10.1002/14651858.CD004667.pub3.

Chapter 7
WIDER EXPERIENCES

Margaret Fisher

Introduction

Midwifery and maternity care specialise in the childbearing period of a woman's life and a neonate's early weeks. Most of your placements will naturally focus on these periods in the continuum of life. What needs to be remembered, however, is that this is only a small part of an individual's journey, and that much may have been happening prior to your involvement in a woman's care and be ongoing throughout this period. This will include physical, psychological and social factors – all of which can have an impact on her pregnancy and childbirth and vice versa.

Although childbearing is essentially a normal physiological process – see the International Confederation of Midwives (ICM) Position Statement on 'Keeping Birth Normal' (ICM 2008, p 1) as discussed in Chapter 5 – this is not always the case. It is worth looking at the information in the National Institute for Health and Care Excellence guidelines and care pathways on 'Antenatal Care' (NICE 2011a), 'Pregnancy and Complex Social Factors' (NICE 2010) and

'Antenatal and Postnatal Mental Health' (NICE 2007) which identify the range of issues that may complicate childbearing. The recent 'Mothers and Babies: Reducing Risk through Audits and Confidential Enquiries across the UK' (MBRRACE-UK 2014) report highlights just how important knowledge of pre-existing medical or mental health conditions is, as 68% of the maternal deaths in the period 2009–2012 were a result of co-existing disorders in pregnancy. When things are not totally straightforward in your career as a midwife, you will be glad of any knowledge and experience that you may have previously gained which will help inform your decisions and actions. Of course, many of these will be acquired in your regular placements and theoretical elements of your pre-registration course. There will however be some conditions, interventions, situations and experiences which may be only rarely or never encountered during your maternity placements. It is wise to make best use of every opportunity as a student to expand your knowledge base whilst you are supernumerary, under the supervision of a registered practitioner

The Hands-on Guide to Midwifery Placements, First Edition.
Edited by Luisa Cescutti-Butler and Margaret Fisher.
© 2016 John Wiley & Sons, Ltd. Published 2016 by John Wiley & Sons, Ltd.

and expected to have learning objectives. You may therefore find it beneficial to consider whether there are any experiences to be gained which may not naturally occur within your existing placements, but which would be useful for your future practice as a midwife. Some of you will have entered your midwifery programme via the shortened route, already being registered nurses. You will find that previous experiences will be invaluable, but you are also encouraged to consider how you could supplement these as you embrace this new career pathway.

The European Union (EU) Directive 2013/35/EU of the European Parliament and of the Council (2013) requires pre-registration midwifery students throughout Europe to gain experience in specific areas which are relevant to their practice:

■ 'Observation and care of the newborn requiring special care including those born pre-term, post-term, underweight or ill.

■ Care of women with pathological conditions in the fields of gynaecology and obstetrics.

■ Initiation into care in the field of medicine and surgery. Initiation shall include theoretical instruction and clinical practice.'

Midwifery programmes vary across the country with respect to how these requirements are addressed and whether or not specific placements outside the usual maternity acute and community areas are part of the formal structure of the curriculum. Inclusion of these in midwifery curricula is largely dependent on the ethos of the programme team and clinical availability. Most programmes will include a focused period gaining experience of gynaecological wards, clinics or theatres as well as a placement in a unit providing specialised care for the neonate (Fig. 7.1-see Chapter 5 which explains the different levels of neonatal facilities provided in Trusts.) The relevance of these placements to midwifery is usually fairly apparent to students. Some programmes may also include allocations to a range of other wards or departments, and students may at first find it difficult to understand why they are being expected to work in an area which does not on the surface appear to be as clearly relevant to midwifery. Medical or surgical wards, emergency departments, intensive care units, theatres and recovery are examples of such placements, as are mental health and outpatient care. Of course, not all patients will be female or of childbearing age – but significant learning can still take place.

The purpose of this chapter is to broaden your awareness of how these wider placements or learning opportunities can provide you with valuable experiences which will contribute to your future care of women and their babies, as well as increasing your understanding of the context of health and social care which surrounds the whole family unit. It is hoped that, through reading this chapter and the vignettes shared by students, you will not only see the benefits of allocated placements but will also feel encouraged to actively seek out additional experiences to address any gaps in your knowledge and skills.

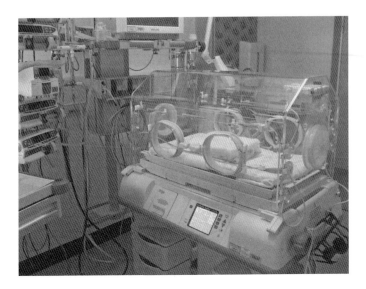

Figure 7.1 Neonatal unit equipment.

Learning opportunities

Midwifery students who have had allocations to wider non-maternity placements describe how learning has been gained not only in specific clinical skills and experiences relevant to the wards or departments but also in role modelling of wider professional factors. Of particular benefit is a broader understanding of the interprofessional environment and teamworking as well as an appreciation of practice and culture in the wider health and social services.

Interprofessional teamworking

Chapter 5 discusses the importance of gaining experience of interprofessional

working and increasing your appreciation of others' roles in the holistic care of women in high-risk situations. Although you will encounter a range of other professionals and support workers in your maternity placements, time spent in other wards or departments will help extend your knowledge and understanding further. You may have the opportunity to work alongside some professionals you have only briefly met or read about in a referral letter. You will experience different teams working in different ways – and there will be positive and weaker examples of how these function, all of which will contribute to your learning. Get as involved as possible in the team, and take every opportunity you can to shadow professionals or follow the care pathways of individual patients.

Attend any team debriefing meetings that are available – particularly if you have been in an area which is very stressful such as Intensive Therapy/Care Unit or Emergency Department. Many midwifery students have particularly valued the support and learning opportunities these have provided.

Communication and interpersonal skills

You will of course encounter communication in every placement and situation during your programme and – as indicated in the Essential Skill Clusters for midwifery (NMC 2009) – this is paramount in your professional practice. Placements in areas other than maternity will likewise provide valuable additional experiences of interprofessional interactions as well as those between carer and client. You may gain some particularly helpful experiences of more complex communication which you may have encountered less frequently in the maternity settings, such as the breaking of bad news.

Kerry Coleman shares with you some very meaningful learning around communication she gained when on placement in the Intensive Care Unit in Vignette 7.1. Read her fourth paragraph that describes how she learned hugely valuable tips about verbal and non-verbal communication which could be directly transferable to her midwifery practice. In contrast, some students have found that – due to the busyness of the environment and different context of care – interprofessional communication in some areas has not been as strong as it should be. There is positive learning to be gained from this too.

Caring for the sick, elderly or dying will also help you to develop your communication skills as you observe others' interactions and 'live' the experience with the patient and their family. Some of these experiences may be challenging for you on a personal level, but if you keep the patient at the centre (just as you do in midwifery), you will find that you can enhance their care as well as extending your own skills to take back to your practice. Demonstrate compassion at all times, remembering that this is one of the vital '6C's' (DoH 2012).

Clinical skills

Chapter 5 discussed the importance of using wider opportunities to learn and practise core clinical skills, as these are needed on both antenatal and postnatal wards as well as during many higher risk labours. If you have a placement on a ward in a non-maternity setting, make good use of this additional range of learning opportunities which will be available, including the following:

- Medicine rounds

- Doctor rounds

- Wound care – dressings, drains, suture and clip removal

- Urinary catheter care – various sites

- Intravenous therapy management

- Clinical observations

- Blanket baths and pressure area care

Vignette 7.1 Emergency department and intensive care unit experiences

'The non-maternity placements allowed me to appreciate how healthy the majority of our service users are and taught me basic nursing care when caring for those who aren't. I was excited about my non-maternity placements and although I had set myself learning objectives, I kept open-minded to new experiences. As a student I have been faced with some unusual scenarios which qualified midwives said they had "never come across in their 40 years as a midwife", including a postnatal mother suffering a stroke and a woman who attended a minor injuries unit with abdominal pains, who turned out to be in labour and the nurse had sought our assistance. I considered what new experiences I was likely to encounter on my non-maternity placements and how they could relate to midwifery, such as caring for the dying or deceased and their families, delivering bad news, emergency management of a clinical condition and effective multidisciplinary working.

Whilst on the Emergency Department, I ensured I stayed with a woman having a stroke and accompanied her through the initial management. I discussed my previous experience with the doctors and nurses and they informed me of "what we can do" in identifying a stroke and the initial time-critical management of their care. Whilst on the Emergency Department I was also honoured when nurses and doctors asked me for guidance on women who arrived in early pregnancy. This made me feel like a valued member of the team – despite only spending a short time here.

My placement on the Intensive Care Unit enabled me to watch a person become acutely unwell – subtle signs, which could be so easily missed, provide vital clues that something is wrong – and as a midwife, it is imperative we are attentive to these signs. The elderly gentleman was thought to be improving, however rapidly became unwell within a 10 minute period. His continuous monitoring showed a rapid development of tachypnoea, tachycardia and hypotension whilst upon observation he appeared pale and clammy. Within maternity, continuous monitoring is not used on women and therefore it is vital we are mindful of these other signs, as this will often be our first warning sign that something is not right. I discussed the scenario with an anaesthetist who supported my feelings and highlighted that the healthy young women we see in maternity often become compromised until the condition is life threatening before displaying these signs and symptoms.

Also, whilst on the Intensive Care Unit, I learnt to care for the family in addition to the patient and became aware that they are often silently observing your actions and interpreting them. For example, your facial expression or "the look" professionals give one another when something isn't going well is picked up by families and can cause them anxiety. I have since adapted my practice and been open and honest with women and their families, sharing information about their situation and whether something is not going to plan or requires immediate

(continued)

intervention. Furthermore, I attended a discussion with a family regarding withdrawing treatment and allowing a gentleman to die peacefully. I discussed the issue of delivering bad news with the consultant and he gave me some useful tips: Be clear and concise, use appropriate terminology such as "death" or "die" as vocabulary such as "passing on" can be misinterpreted, deliver the important information within the first two sentences as people will not listen beyond this, go the extra mile in having knowledge about the future and support services that are available.

I have thoroughly enjoyed all of my non-maternity placements and I feel they have enhanced my skills as a midwife. It is important to make the most of these non-maternity placements as it is unlikely that we will ever have this opportunity during our working careers!'

Kerry Coleman
Third-year student, Plymouth University, Devon, UK
Reproduced with permission of Kerry Coleman

- Infection control procedures

- Lifting and handling

- Bed-making, ward hygiene and serving meals.

You will learn much by working alongside nurses as they undertake medicine rounds of a far more comprehensive nature than you will experience in midwifery, and this will stand you in good stead for your future practice. Gill Gosling's experience in Vignette 7.2 is an example of this. You will have the chance to learn about a greater range of drugs and their indications and side effects and will also benefit in practising administration through a variety of routes. Please ensure local policies are followed at all times and you are under direct supervision of a registered professional throughout.

In the same way, you are likely to have the opportunity to be involved in dressings and other surgical devices which will prepare you well for any

post-operative care you encounter in your midwifery profession. It will also enhance your dexterity and reinforce the principles of infection control.

Try to work alongside support workers such as care assistants or Band 4 staff. Maternity support workers provide a very valuable role in the maternity care team, but increased reliance on these colleagues to provide what used to be within the midwife's remit has resulted in decreased opportunities for midwifery students to learn and practise the basic clinical and caring skills. The recent findings of the Francis Report, Morecambe Bay and Keogh Reports (DoH 2013; NMC 2012; NHS England 2013) amongst others have been sobering in their condemnation of unsatisfactory levels of basic care across health professions and clinical specialities. Use these placements to get to grips with what is extremely important learning.

You may have an opportunity to be placed in more specialist departments;

'When it comes to medicines and the way in which they work, the majority of people either find them easy to pick up or a complete challenge! Personally, I find medications very interesting and as a result find them relatively easy to remember.

When on placement, I have a habit of collecting the information sheets from inside the medicine boxes so that I have a record of medications I have seen given; if I do this, then I am more likely to remember what it was used for if it comes up again.

One of the most memorable occasions, for me, relating to medication is when I was asked to give vitamin B12 injections under direct supervision of my mentor. I did not know what the injection was for or how many the woman would require so I asked my mentor. My mentor was not certain on the specifics of the drug, so we looked it up in the BNF – there were several drug regimes listed. The prescription was checked with a senior obstetrician and eventually with a consultant haematologist. It turned out that the woman was receiving an appropriate course of treatment, however until this was clarified, neither my mentor nor I was happy to administer the treatment.

This was a valuable learning experience and it taught me to question regimes/medication if they are not familiar and to seek advice from appropriate sources – whether that is the BNF or specialist consultants.

The hospital I trained in did not do formal drug rounds, so I found it very helpful to do these on my non-maternity placements.'

Gill Gosling
Third-year student, Plymouth University, Devon, UK
Reproduced with permission of Gill Gosling

the next section in this chapter will identify some of the specific clinical skills you may learn in these areas.

Learning about conditions

As discussed in Chapter 5, any opportunity to learn more about medical or mental health conditions is to be grasped. If you are placed in non-maternity areas, you will be able to gain experiences which may not be the norm in a midwifery setting, but which will provide you with increased confidence should you encounter these in future practice. The recent MBRRACE-UK report (2014) demonstrates clearly the contribution of pre-existing or new medical or mental health conditions to the morbidity and mortality of childbearing women and their babies. It is therefore evident that a deeper understanding of these conditions – the causes, detection, management and prevention – is needed. 'Think Sepsis' is one of the key topic-specific messages for care in this report.

Recognition of deterioration and an understanding of the actions to take and referral pathways to follow is a 'must'. Women who may not previously have been able to conceive are now increasingly having successful pregnancies, but these may be putting the woman's own health in jeopardy and she will need careful monitoring. Women you encounter in midwifery practice may have coagulation or metabolic disorders, suffer from epilepsy or cardiac problems. Cardiac disease is currently the leading indirect cause of maternal death (MBRRACE-UK 2014). Women with congenital disorders such as cystic fibrosis are living longer and becoming mothers themselves. Diabetes and hypertension are on the increase. Some women for whom you care may have cancer. An understanding of the impact of pregnancy and childbirth on these conditions as well as of the condition on the maternal or fetal health is essential. You may well learn about some of these complications during your taught sessions, but nothing quite replaces the experience of sharing part of a patient's journey and being exposed to the reality of diagnosis and treatment.

You are encouraged to read up on any conditions which present in your daily work within your midwifery placements. This will help you to better appreciate the implications and understand the management. These opportunities will, however, be limited – and so a proactive approach to embracing any occasions when you may encounter these in non-maternity settings is essential. You need to step outside the box of thinking that you will only learn if you are in a midwifery setting. If you attend a respiratory clinic and participate in a consultation with an elderly man with asthma, transfer this new knowledge to women you book in the antenatal period with this condition. An appreciation of the impact of haemorrhage and hypertensive disorders on the body systems can be gained through experiences of caring for other patient groups and easily translated to midwifery practice. Observing a woman having a mastectomy will teach you much about surgical procedures, breast anatomy and the implications of cancer for individuals. A young man in pain needs as much support as a woman in labour, and caring for an elderly woman with a prolapsed uterus will show you the reality of the outcome of trauma in childbirth or inadequate pelvic floor exercises.

Opportunities to be involved in resuscitation, care of the dying and last rites in a setting outside the maternity environment will also provide invaluable learning which – although every midwife hopes s/he will never need to use this – will enhance your knowledge, teamworking and clinical skills as well as help you to learn coping strategies and interpersonal skills which will be of enormous benefit in your future practice. Make sure you are well supported at the time and afterwards if this occurs; as previously stated, students have often found this to be a particular strength in areas where these events are not unusual occurrences.

Specific learning

In Plymouth University – as in some others – we have a long track record of including focused non-maternity placements in our pre-registration programme. The 'destinations' have been modified over the years in response to student feedback about their learning as well as service changes, but they have continued to form an essential element of the programme. Many midwives who qualified elsewhere have commented that they wished they had also benefitted from these experiences during their training. Figure 7.2 indicates key learning common to all areas, which midwifery students have found of particular value over the years. In Boxes 7.1–7.6, you will find some examples of specific learning relevant to particular placements. Some of these are drawn from a local evaluation project (Fisher 2006) while others have been identified by students anecdotally or through their written accounts of their experiences. You will recall Kerry's reflection on the experiences she gained in her Emergency Department and Intensive Care Unit placements in Vignette 7.1. Now read Mollie Craig's account of the beneficial learning she achieved in her Gynaecology placement in Vignette 7.3.

Although your programme may not include formal allocations to these areas, it is highly likely that you will be able to negotiate 'ad hoc' experiences in specific clinics or departments, or that other

---

Vignette 7.3   Gynaecology placement learning

'After this placement, I feel that my nursing skills have improved. I learnt things that I hadn't seen in midwifery which was beneficial even if it wasn't directly relevant, such as assessment of pressure sores and comfort rounds. My knowledge of early pregnancy has increased through time on the early pregnancy unit and viewing early ultrasound scans and dating scans. I hope that this knowledge will enhance my midwifery practice such as problems encountered when booking a woman in the community, as well as understanding conditions when I see them in a woman's history. I feel my knowledge of gynaecological conditions has improved dramatically. This will enable me to care better for women who have existing gynaecological conditions such as fibroids. I will also understand the treatment better as well as the pathology of the conditions. This will be beneficial when booking in the community and during labour when the birth plan may need to be adjusted to accommodate care of the gynaecological condition. The ward rounds with the doctors were very beneficial to observe. It was good to learn about the treatment and symptoms of the conditions. This may help me to be more wary of certain conditions women may be suffering from, as it may indicate an underlying gynaecological condition.'

Mollie Craig
Second-year student, Plymouth University, Devon, UK
Reproduced with permission of Mollie Craig

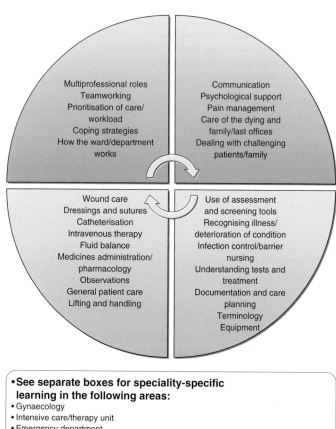

Multiprofessional roles
Teamworking
Prioritisation of care/
workload
Coping strategies
How the ward/department
works

Communication
Psychological support
Pain management
Care of the dying and
family/last offices
Dealing with challenging
patients/family

Wound care
Dressings and sutures
Catheterisation
Intravenous therapy
Fluid balance
Medicines administration/
pharmacology
Observations
General patient care
Lifting and handling

Use of assessment
and screening tools
Recognising illness/
deterioration of condition
Infection control/barrier
nursing
Understanding tests and
treatment
Documentation and care
planning
Terminology
Equipment

- **See separate boxes for speciality-specific
  learning in the following areas:**
  - Gynaecology
  - Intensive care/therapy unit
  - Emergency department
  - Theatres and recovery
  - Medical wards/departments
  - Neonatal units

Figure 7.2 Key learning in non-maternity settings.

health or social care professionals will be happy for you to spend a day or so shadowing them. A short time spent in a high dependency area such as an intensive care/therapy unit could be very beneficial as the MBRRACE-UK report (2014) identifies the need for there to be adequate provision of appropriate critical care facilities for women even on delivery suites – so some familiarity with an area such as this could prove useful in your future career. Talk to your personal tutor or mentor to find out whether and how this can be arranged, remembering that students from other professions will also need to access these experiences. This will help you to achieve your EU requirements as well as provide a more rounded knowledge and skills base from which you can draw in your future career. Be creative and proactive, and you will reap the benefits. Sara Evans describes in detail how valuable she found a focused experience of the Fertility Unit during her elective period in Chapter 8. You could perhaps arrange a similar 'ad hoc' experience either earlier in your programme or in your own 'Staycation' elective option.

Box 7.1   Gynaecology

■ Understanding where maternity and gynaecology take over from each other.

■ Impact of childbearing on later life events and preventative care/treatment (e.g. bladder and pelvic floor).

■ Experience of pregnancy disorders – ectopic pregnancy and hyperemesis.

■ Pre- and post-operative care, including following a woman throughout her experience.

■ Gynaecology surgery/theatre experience.

■ Day case unit.

■ Clinics, for example colposcopy, genito-urinary medicine (GUM), fertility, termination of pregnancy, female genital mutilation (FGM) and post-menopausal bleeding.

■ Early pregnancy screening and ultrasound scans.

■ Providing emotional support to patients with cancer and other serious illnesses.

■ Assisting patients with physical disabilities.

■ Epidural management.

■ Bladder scanning.

■ Doctor rounds and ward work.

Box 7.2 Intensive care/therapy unit

■ Criteria for admission.

■ Care of medical/surgical/paediatric emergency.

■ Care pathway of obstetric disorders/related disorders.

■ Preparation of women for what they may experience (e.g., noise of monitors and one-to-one care).

■ Care of the unconscious/intubated patient; maintenance of airway.

■ Resuscitation.

■ Care of the extremely ill patient.

■ Involvement of family in care provision.

■ Problem-solving to meet needs of patients and family.

■ Understanding of body systems and responses to illnesses.

■ Multi-organ failure and hypovolaemic shock.

■ Heart rate patterns.

■ Inserting naso-gastric tube.

■ Observation of pressure area care.

■ Central Venous Pressure monitoring.

■ Importance of identification (e.g. patient label and line identity).

Box 7.3 Emergency department

■ Resuscitation.

■ Electrocardiography (ECG), rhythm, anatomy and physiology of the heart.

■ Triage.

■ Identifying people who are becoming ill/deterioration in condition.

■ Recognising signs of shock.

■ Glasgow Coma Scale/neurological observations.

- Care of medical/surgical/orthopaedic/paediatric emergency.

- Care of minor injuries.

- Seeing CT scans.

- Reading X-rays.

- Plastering and slings.

- Observation of treatment of children, men and the elderly.

- Gynaecological problems (ectopic, miscarriage with arterial bleed, post-operative bleed).

- Attending specialist areas and clinics, for example eye room, asthma clinic, diabetic clinic, DVT clinic and walk-in centre.

- Developing interview skills.

Box 7.4 Theatres and recovery

- Pre and post-operative care.

- Following through a patient in theatre, recovery, transfer to ward.

- Intubation and airway management.

- Management of the unconscious patient.

- Immediate post-operative wound and intravenous therapy management.

- Anaesthetic administration – general, epidural, spinal and local.

- Aseptic and sterile procedures.

- Pain response and management.

- Signs of shock, haemorrhage, deterioration.

- Anatomical learning while observing surgery.

- Surgical procedures.

Box 7.5 Medical wards/departments

■ Attending clinics linked to ward and at GP surgeries – for example, asthma, diabetic, thyroid, cardiac, angioplasty, dermatology, pain management, DVT, chest and tissue viability.

■ Management of medical conditions – for example, diabetes and monitoring/insulin regimes, hypertension, asthma and other chest complaints, renal failure/function/haemodialysis, cardiac problems, dermatology, cancer and anaemia.

■ Visiting other areas associated with ward – for example, outpatients, radiography and acute medical admissions.

■ Care of stroke patients and rehabilitation.

■ Dealing with dementia and care of the elderly.

■ Tests and investigations – for example, electrocardiographs (ECG), spirometry, lumbar puncture, X-rays, CT scan, CPAP/ventilators, endoscopy, kidney biopsy and sleep studies.

■ Renal dialysis.

■ Chemotherapy.

■ Use of oxygen.

■ Managing sepsis.

■ MRSA awareness, barrier and reverse barrier nursing/infection control/closed ward protocols.

■ Blood transfusions.

■ Sample collection.

■ History taking.

■ Preventing pressure sores.

■ Personal hygiene and use of commode.

■ Assessment/planning/implementing/evaluating care using care plan and nursing notes (i.e. nursing process).

■ Holistic care of patients and relatives.

■ Sociology – sick role and medical model.

■ Health education and health promotion.

Box 7.6 Neonatal units

■ Intensive, high dependency, special or transitional care.

■ Knowledge of procedures and equipment to be able to share with women and their partners/understand what they are experiencing if their baby is on the neonatal unit.

■ Health education, health promotion and developmental care.

■ Case conferences/social service involvement.

■ Neonatal resuscitation – in real life or teaching parents.

■ Readmission to the neonatal unit for weight loss management.

■ The importance of preventing preterm labour due to the health risks to the neonate.

■ Care of the preterm neonate including initiation of breastfeeding and kangaroo care.

■ Neonatal jaundice – causes, identification, levels and treatment.

■ Recognition and care of the sick term neonate.

■ Airway management and use of oxygen.

■ Fluid balance and nutrition in the neonate.

■ Thermoregulation.

■ Managing sepsis.

■ Drug withdrawal.

■ Monitors and equipment.

■ Sample collection.

■ Transportation of the neonate from labour ward to the neonatal unit, or to other hospitals.

Other useful experiences

Mental health

Some midwifery programmes may include a placement in an area of the mental health services. This is perhaps less commonly the case as these are very specialist and it is not always appropriate to have visiting students. There should, however, be some facility in your area in which you can gain some experience in this increasingly important aspect of care.

The National Institute for Health and Care Excellence guidelines and clinical pathways on mental health (NICE 2007, 2011b, 2014) make it very clear how much a part of midwifery practice this is becoming. The MBRRACE-UK report (2014) identifies that mental conditions remain an important indirect cause of maternal death. Changes in the structure and functioning of society, dependence on damaging substances and psychological stressors can all contribute to mental health problems. It would therefore be beneficial for you to gain as much experience in this area as possible; some suggestions are below. You may be able to work alongside some of these professionals, or at least arrange a meeting with them to discuss their role and the links with maternal mental health. Find out about the availability of wider mental health facilities in your area too:

■ Specialist midwives (mental health, drugs and alcohol)

■ Perinatal Mental Health Team, if your Trust has this service

■ Mother and Baby Unit, if there is one in the area

■ Inpatient psychiatry team

■ Psychiatrist

■ Community psychiatric nurse

■ Perinatal infant mental health specialist

■ Access and well-being/other assessment and community support

■ Crisis/emergency team

■ Recovery/independent living/longer term care provision

■ Drugs/alcohol rehabilitation services

■ Safeguarding and vulnerable adults

■ Mental health disorders

■ Triage and referral

■ Process for sectioning under the Mental Health Act.

Other departments

Don't forget that maternity care, along with all direct clinical services, relies on the support of many wider departments. These facilities may be found in either hospital or community settings. Try to find opportunity to visit some of the following:

■ Pharmacy (Fig. 7.3)

■ Pathology laboratory

■ Haematology

■ Blood bank/blood transfusion service

■ Physiotherapy department

■ Dietetics department

■ X-ray department

■ Nuclear medicine department

■ Records department

■ Registrar's office

■ Chaplaincy

■ Children's centres/Surestart

■ Clubs/groups/workshops (e.g. baby/breastfeeding/church/community/pregnancy yoga/active birth)

■ Craniopathy/acupuncture/alternative therapy clinic

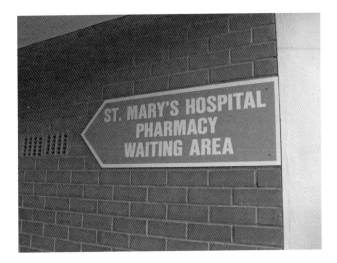

Figure 7.3 Pharmacy.

How to prepare

Although there is much valuable learning to be gained, you also need to be aware of some of the challenges which are not uncommon in these non-maternity areas so that you are prepared for them. These may include the following:

■ Not being expected.

■ Not feeling welcomed.

■ Lack of continuity of 'mentorship' (or no specific individual identified for support).

■ Staff not knowing why midwifery students are there.

■ Staff not knowing midwifery students' capabilities or having unrealistic expectations of them (comparing them with nursing students at the same stage, or not recognising additional skills such as venepuncture).

■ Students not knowing about available learning opportunities or having unrealistic expectations of the placement.

■ Students not seeing the 'bigger picture' and therefore finding it difficult to apply experiences to the midwifery context.

■ Students not wanting to attend – not seeing the relevance or thinking they are missing valuable 'midwifery' experiences/ pressure of meeting programme or EU requirements/not wanting to work in an unfamiliar environment.

Clearly, some of these are outside your control, but you have a part to play in reducing many of these challenges. If you want to make best use of your experience – whether structured or 'ad hoc' – some key actions will improve your chances of looking back on this as a positive learning experience. Many of these have already been included in other chapters, as they are of course relevant to all placements. The evaluation project at Plymouth University (Fisher and Arkinstall 2006) which focused specifically on non-maternity placements identified *The 5 P's of Successful Placements* on which this guidance is based:

1 *Preparation*

■ Use your practice portfolio to identify gaps in knowledge/skills and areas needing development.

■ Seek advice from your personal tutor/ academic advisor or the University placements team for further information.

■ Contact the clinical area, department or individual professional – phone or visit. This shows interest, confirms attendance, increases the likelihood of your being allocated a designated mentor or supervisor for the experience and enables you to negotiate shifts.

■ Ask if the area has any induction/ information packs or details about specific learning opportunities which may be available.

■ Complete any preparatory packs the area may provide.

■ Identify specific learning objectives for the placement or day, drawing from all of the above.

2 *Planning*

■ On the first day of your placement, discuss your learning objectives with your designated mentor or an interested staff member. Identify any additional experiences they may guide you towards which may be particularly relevant to the area. This will help them to understand the purpose of your placement as well as demonstrate your willingness to learn.

■ Discuss and plan any specific activities (e.g. visits to clinics or other departments, shadowing other health professionals).

■ Be prepared to be flexible.

3 *Participation*

■ You are far more likely to get a friendly response and your questions answered if you show an interest and enthusiasm.

■ Be open to other views and willing to learn from all categories of staff. Respect individuals and their roles.

■ Be prepared to work as part of the team – help them and they will help you.

■ Although it is likely you will spend some of the time observing, be prepared to take part as much as possible.

■ Don't consider any task too menial or irrelevant – the basics are extremely important and learning is to be gained from all situations.

4 *Punctuality*

■ Make sure your shift commitments are clear and that you attend all – on time.

■ If for any reason you are unable to attend, communicate appropriately with the clinical area and University, following local policy.

■ Try to make up missed time during the placement period, if at all possible; you may otherwise not be able to achieve all your learning objectives.

5 *Positive approach*

■ Relate your experiences to your midwifery practice as far as possible – remember that the people you care for do not necessarily have to be female or pregnant in order for you to learn from the situation.

- A positive approach will achieve the most learning for you and help to make the placement an enjoyable experience for everyone.

- You are having the opportunity to see a different approach to health care and to learn valuable skills. Once you are a qualified midwife, you are unlikely to have these opportunities again – so make the most of them.

Gill's summary of 'Preparing for non-maternity placements' in Vignette 7.4 confirms these principles from her own experience over the last 3 years, and further 'top tips' can be seen in Box 7.7.

Conclusion

I hope that this chapter will have inspired you to make best use of any opportunities you may have for wider learning in non-maternity settings. These may be a structured component of your programme or 'ad hoc' experiences you have sought to address yourself. You are strongly encouraged to be proactive in identifying gaps in your knowledge and skills to seek out the best ways of 'closing the loop' in whatever ways your programme, institution or clinical environment allows. Use any flexible periods, draw on other professionals' expertise and be prepared to move out of your comfort zone in order to make you a more rounded, knowledgeable and confident midwife.

In conclusion, let past students speak to you from their own experiences. Thanks go to the anonymous contributors from the evaluation project (Fisher and Arkinstall 2006) who wrote the illuminating comments shown in Fig. 7.4:

"Nursing care is different to midwifery and if that concept is accepted by the student then it should be a very important and positive experience – midwifery and pregnancy is only one part of the larger picture of women's health."

"It helped me to think in a wider way about aspects of care that I think you could easily miss out on when you don't have a nursing background, and it is good to clarify that although we deal with (on the whole) healthy young women, the health promotion we give can benefit in later life."

"I feel I learnt to understand why people get agitated about being in hospital, and I feel I learnt that communication skills are vitally important in dealing with these situations, often defusing problems just by acknowledging worries."

"I learnt more about diabetes by going to the diabetes centre clinic for 4 hours than I feel I have learnt in 2 years of my training! Although we learn about the physiology of diabetes, the theory does not teach us about the person behind the disease and how they manage their condition day to day."

"They have a very busy unit and are keen to involve students in all aspects of care from drug rounds to assisting consultants – who are also keen to teach, but the student must be aware of what is happening and ask to be involved. I was never turned down."

"Made me think deeply about myself and how I wanted to practice. I began to feel the responsibility of the midwife compared to what I saw as the responsibilities of the nurse."

"I gave a foot massage to a lady who needed cream rubbing into her heels; no one had done this for days. As we chatted the old lady cried because she was so lonely and was touched by someone giving her the time to talk. It was a really enriching experience, and I shall take this back to midwifery practice. It's the small things that, basic caring and listening one to one, that matter."

Figure 7.4 What students have said about their experiences in non-maternity settings.

Box 7.7 Top Tips

■ Be prepared to move out of your comfort zone.

■ Find out about available opportunities – talk to fellow students, academic or clinical staff, service users.

■ Use the expertise of others – shadow other health or social care professionals/specialists.

■ Arrange observational visits or tours (e.g. pharmacy, laboratory, council registrar, outpatients departments and clinics).

■ Prepare yourself and the receiving practitioner or clinical area for your visit.

■ Don't be narrow-minded – lots can be learned irrespective of the client's age, gender or environment.

■ Read around experiences gained to reinforce learning and apply this to the midwifery context.

■ Make the most of these opportunities during your programme – once you are a registered midwife, they will be much more limited.

And from fellow Plymouth University students, Kerry Coleman (third year) and Keri Morter (second year):

■ Be open minded.

■ Have a positive attitude and show this whilst on placement.

■ Actively seek experiences whilst there.

■ Ask questions and make the most of having access to professionals with lots of experience within the area.

■ The harder you work and the more interested you are, the more you will learn; use your initiative once you start to get an understanding of things and offer to do tasks you are competent in such as observations, before you are asked.

■ Every experience can relate to midwifery somehow – even though it may not seem like it does at the time.

References

Department of Health (2012) Compassion in practice: nursing, midwifery and care staff – our vision and strategy. Available at http://www.england.nhs.uk/wp-content/uploads/2012/12/compassion-in-practice.pdf (last accessed 30 July 2014).

Department of Health (2013) Report of the Mid Staffordshire NHS Foundation Trust Public Inquiry (Francis Report). The Stationery Office Limited, London. Available at http://www.midstaffspublicinquiry.com/sites/default/files/report/Executive%20summary.pdf (last accessed 1 August 2014).

European Parliament (2013) Recognition of professional qualifications. Available at http://ec.europa.eu/internal_market/qualifications/policy_developments/legislation/index_en.htm (last accessed 29 July 2014).

Fisher M and Arkinstall T (2006) *Report on Evaluation of Non-maternity Placements for Midwifery Students 2004–2006*. Plymouth University, Plymouth.

International Confederation of Midwives (2008) Position Statement: Keeping Birth Normal. Available at http://internationalmidwives.org/assets/uploads/documents/Position%20Statements%20-%20English/PS2008_007%20ENG%20Keeping%20Birth%20Normal.pdf (last accessed 28 July 2014).

Mothers and Babies: Reducing Risk through Audits and Confidential Enquiries across the UK (MBRRACE-UK) (2014) *Saving Lives, Improving Mothers' Care*. National Perinatal Epidemiology Unit, Oxford. Available at https://www.npeu.ox.ac.uk/downloads/files/mbrrace-uk/reports/Saving%20Lives%20Improving%20Mothers%20Care%20report%202014%20Full.pdf (last accessed 24 February 2015).

National Health Service England (2013) Review into the quality of care and treatment provided by 14 hospital Trusts in England: overview report (Keogh Report). Available at http://www.nhs.uk/NHSEngland/bruce-keogh-review/Documents/outcomes/keogh-review-final-report.pdf (last accessed 1 August 2014).

National Institute for Health and Care Excellence (2007) Antenatal and postnatal mental health (NICE Guideline CG45). Available at http://www.nice.org.uk/guidance/CG45 (last accessed 31 July 2014).

National Institute for Health and Care Excellence (2010) Pregnancy and complex social factors: a model for service provision for pregnant women with complex social factors (NICE Guideline CG110). Available at http://www.nice.org.uk/guidance/CG110 (last accessed 31 July 2014).

National Institute for Health and Care Excellence (2011a) Antenatal care pathway. Available at http://pathways.nice.org.uk/pathways/antenatal-care (last accessed 31 July 2014).

National Institute for Health and Care Excellence (2011b) Common mental health disorders: identification and pathways to care (NICE Guideline CG123). Available at http://www.nice.org.uk/guidance/CG123 (last accessed 31 July 2014).

National Institute for Health and Care Excellence (2014) Antenatal and postnatal mental health pathway. Available at http://pathways.nice.org.uk/pathways/antenatal-and-postnatal-mental-health?fno=1# (last accessed 31 July 2014).

Nursing and Midwifery Council (2009) *Standards for pre-registration midwifery education*. Nursing and Midwifery Council, London. Available at http://www.nmc-uk.org/Documents/NMC-Publications/nmcStandardsforPre_RegistrationMidwiferyEducation.pdf (last accessed 28 July 2014).

Nursing and Midwifery Council (2012) *Nursing and Midwifery Council of University Hospitals of Morecambe Bay NHS Foundation Trust*. Nursing and Midwifery Council, London.

Available at http://www.nmc-uk.org/Documents/MidwiferyExtraordinaryReviewReports/Final%20Morecambe%20Bay%20extra%20ordinary%20report%2020120907.pdf (last accessed 1 August 2014).

Further resources

Centre for Maternal and Child Enquiries (CMACE) reports: http://www.hqip.org.uk/cmace-reports/.

General Medical Council (GMC): www.gmc-uk.org.

Health and Care Professions Council (HCPC): www.hcpc-uk.org.uk.

Mothers and babies: reducing risk through audits and confidential enquiries across the UK (MBRRACE-UK): https://www.npeu.ox.ac.uk/mbrrace-uk.

National Institute for Health and Care Excellence (NICE): www.nice.org.uk.

Royal College of Anaesthetists: www.rcoa.ac.uk.

Royal College of Nursing: www.rcn.org.uk.

Royal College of Obstetricians and Gynaecologists: www.rcog.org.uk.

Royal College of Paediatricians: www.rcpch.ac.uk.

Royal College of Physicians: www.rcplondon.ac.uk.

Royal College of Psychiatrists: www.rcpsych.ac.uk.

Royal College of Surgeons: www.rcseng.ac.uk.

Chapter 8
STUDENT ELECTIVES

Luisa Cescutti-Butler

Introduction

'Dear students

I have made contact with a midwifery lecturer in Johannesburg, South Africa, who will be able to arrange an elective for two students in July, there is some flexibility around this. Please see an extract of what you may be able to do whilst over there . . . '

is an outline of an email sent to third-year midwifery students, concerning an elective placement overseas. Silvia's response

'My concern is the costs and how to finance this trip. I am not sure how much/if the University would provide any financial help, that is what worries me.'

raises some of the issues students are typically faced with when considering undertaking an elective overseas to experience midwifery within a global context.

As student midwives, you may have an opportunity during your training to undertake an elective placement that could be in another hospital within the location of your University's placement areas, maternity hospitals within the United Kingdom or abroad, to observe midwifery in different and in some cases challenging healthcare settings. Wherever you decide to go, or whatever you decide to do, this chapter will help focus your thinking by considering the following issues:

- What is an elective placement?

- Reasons for undertaking an elective.

- Planning for the elective experience:

- What could you do in this period?

- Planning your expenses.

- Practicalities.

- What next?

What is an elective placement?

The elective period, which usually takes place in the third year of your midwifery programme, provides you with an opportunity to observe midwifery and in some cases non-midwifery practice in

---

The Hands-on Guide to Midwifery Placements, First Edition.
Edited by Luisa Cescutti-Butler and Margaret Fisher.
© 2016 John Wiley & Sons, Ltd. Published 2016 by John Wiley & Sons, Ltd.

different healthcare settings (see Chapter 7 for more information about the latter). You may choose to stay within your local area or select an institution within the United Kingdom to visit or travel abroad somewhere; universities may offer different options. Many students elect to use this time to experience midwifery care in settings other than the National Health Service (NHS) such as independent midwifery (more on this later). These learning opportunities are not normally available during your educational programme, and it is therefore an ideal time for you to explore a variety of experiences. Some students, however, simply choose a more practical approach and undertake electives in areas where there may be future employment prospects.

How long are elective placements?

Elective placement lengths vary, generally ranging from a 2- to 4-week period, and up to 12 weeks in some universities. For example, midwifery students at Plymouth University (PU) undertake an elective placement of 4 weeks, and Bournemouth University (BU) students have an elective which lasts 12 weeks, starting in June of their third year.

Reasons for undertaking an elective

Firstly, it can broaden your midwifery skills, knowledge and experience. Depending on where you to choose to go, you may elect to extend your

understanding around diversity of childbirth by experiencing midwifery practice in different birth settings (Wilson 2014). Not only will you be developing a new set of skills, but you will also be able to contribute to the learning environment. In turn, this will extend your interpersonal skills and boost your confidence, especially if you are away from the security of your normal placement area (Wilson 2014). Secondly, if you choose to go abroad, you will be able to experience cultures and practices different from your own and observe how healthcare is delivered in countries where resources may be lacking (Einterz 2008). Thirdly, some students would like to work in the charitable sector once qualified and undertaking an elective in a particular area or country will help pave the way for future employment opportunities. Other reasons include some of the following:

■ If you have a particular interest or intend to specialise in an aspect of midwifery, you may be able to 'shadow' specialist midwives which will enable you to enhance your knowledge around your chosen interest, for example Teenage Pregnancy Midwife or Substance Misuse Midwife.

■ Undertake a shortened course (e.g. an introduction to complementary therapies or basic counselling skills) which would enhance your practice as a midwife.

■ Personal and professional development opportunities, providing you with direction for your career and ongoing prospects.

What could you do in this period?

There may be several options available for you to consider:

a. 'Staycation' – remain in your clinical location.

b. 'Staycation with a twist' – remain within the Trusts where your University places midwifery students (Way & Little 2014).

c. UK based but outside the locality of your University placements.

d. Overseas elective.

e. Erasmus Programme.

f. Other ideas/opportunities.

Before deciding on what you would like to do, discuss your ideas with your Personal Tutor (PT) or Academic Assessor (AA) as there may be conditions to be met which are set by your University. These may include the following:

■ Theory and practice for years one and two must be successfully completed.

■ All theoretical learning and assessments completed for third year.

■ All your European Union (EU) requirements (40 births etc.) must be achieved.

■ You may not be able to undertake an elective abroad if you've had an extended period of sickness, especially around the time you submit your application.

If your PT/AA is satisfied you have met the requirements set by your University, you can begin to consider the options available to you. Many universities request elective plans a year in advance of the proposed travel if you are considering an elective abroad. Let's now look at each option in more depth.

'Staycation' – remain in your clinical location

This is where you stay in the clinical hospital where you have undertaken your training. Prior to choosing this option, you will need to identify, in conjunction with your PT/AA, what experience you still need and in which areas this can be achieved. If you have yet to complete the required number of births, you may decide to do a set number of weeks on Labour Ward (LW), but early planning is necessary. You will need to share your proposal with the University placement staff who will liaise with the relevant clinicians (such as the Practice Development Midwife or ward manager) in the area. This is because first- and second-year students will still be having their regular placements, and each ward is only able to take a set number of students per shift. Each placement area will therefore, have to carefully consider your request in combination with overall student numbers to ensure equity of mentoring and experience. Many students choose the 'staycation' option simply because they cannot afford to travel abroad or have family commitments which make it difficult for them to plan a placement that is not local. Staying in the unit where you have trained also enables you to consolidate your practice where the staff know you.

When students were asked what their top tips were for undertaking an elective, one replied

'You don't have to go somewhere exotic for the elective to be interesting and beneficial.'

As the quote suggests, the 'staycation' option is just as valuable provided you have set yourself learning objectives and goals to achieve. Sara Evans from Plymouth University describes how invaluable she found a focused 'staycation' experience of the Fertility Unit during her elective period in Vignette 8.1. You may wish to broaden your knowledge and experience by seeking some of the opportunities Chapter 7 suggests, such as in non-maternity settings. Remember to follow local policy regarding arranging these placements.

Vignette 8.1 Fertility Unit

'During my elective I wanted to concentrate on learning more about IVF (in vitro fertilisation). Fertility treatments are on the increase and I wanted more experience to help me care for women and families who have accessed them.

My first surprise on this placement was being told to not wear any perfume – this is because some chemicals have negative effects on sperm and embryos. Interestingly though, Lily of the Valley perfume can have a positive effect on sperm and fertilisation!

I'm definitely not saying wear Lily of the Valley for this placement – for a start you'd have to wear a huge amount to affect sperm, much more than tolerable. It's just a good example of how sensitive the IVF process is. So, I don't usually wear perfume anyway, but I made sure not to on this placement!

The staff were warm and welcoming. They showed me around the ward and I noticed the calm and quiet atmosphere compared to the main hospital. I was given theatre scrubs and shoes to wear so that I could follow women through their procedures. I shadowed a nurse who met the women on arrival, and she explained that I was a student midwife, and asked them if they would mind me watching the egg collection process. Informed consent was gained without pressure.

I was able to support the women by explaining how to use the gas and air effectively, as egg collection can be an uncomfortable procedure. I was also able to give them some emotional support. I was glad to have these transferable skills from midwifery practice.

The whole theatre team understood that egg collection is a vulnerable, uncomfortable, and important event for women undergoing fertility treatment. Though it takes place in the lithotomy position, privacy and dignity is maintained by having only essential people in theatre. Staff also talked warmly and with respect to the women and families undergoing treatment, explaining the procedure as it progressed.

(continued)

I watched the egg collection on ultrasound, then followed the eggs through to the laboratory where the embryologists examined the samples collected, counted the eggs, and washed and prepared them for fertilisation.

In another laboratory, I was able to look at the sperm samples through the microscope. The embryologist explained the procedure of assessing the quality of the sperm and I was able to see the variety within one sample. Some had two heads or two tails, some were swimming in circles. I was surprised at the low-tech approach to assessing sperm count; the embryologists just use a grid and count the sperm one by one! The samples were cleaned and prepared for fertilisation.

I watched both the IVF and the ICSI (intra-cytoplasmic sperm injection) procedure. I felt privileged to be able to see the exact moment when the sperm was injected into the egg. I felt overwhelmed that this could be a new life – as student midwives we get to see so many awe inspiring events, but the fact that fertilisation usually happens internally, and without even the knowledge of the mother in question, meant this was a special and unusual experience.

I would encourage you to seek out interesting placements. It helped me make sense of theory learnt in year 1 on fertilisation. I find that I learn by doing, and this experience will stay with me throughout my career.

I now feel better able to look after women who have a baby conceived through IVF. I was able to discuss the complex medications and difficult side effects, the emotional and financial difficulties, and invasive procedures, with the women using the service. I now have a greater understanding of women's needs for continuous support and reassurance.'

Sara Evans
Third-year student, Plymouth University
Reproduced with permission of Sara Evans

'Staycation with a twist' – remain within the Trusts where your University places midwifery students

Here you would seek to undertake placements within the locations your University places midwifery students. Universities around the United Kingdom allocate their students to many different clinical sites which may provide various models of midwifery care. It is important that prior to making a decision on where you would like to go, you have researched the other sites within the catchment area of your University. For example, seeking a placement in a clinical site which is very similar to your own may not offer you anything differ... in terms of experience, although each hospital will have slightly different working practices. Taking yourself out of your comfort zone may help to increase your confidence in other ways, such as, if most of your placements have been in an acute hospital which is consultant led, you may choose a locality where birth is entirely facilitated by midwives.

The majority of Becky Fry's training took place in a busy high-risk consultant-led unit and she chose to spend part of her elective in a birth centre where she was able to experience midwives working autonomously including witnessing women birthing physiologically. Working within this environment also provided her with additional skills around risk assessment and decision-making. Here follows an extract of her experience:

'I chose to work within settings which are led in a variety of ways different to the Trust in which I trained. I wanted to experience the environments and attitudes of care staff as well as meet service users from a variety of socio-economic groups. With the majority of my training taking place in a busy high risk consultant led unit, I wanted to experience the autonomy of the midwives in a birth centre along with witnessing normal physiological birth, gaining additional skills in risk assessing and decision making. Another Trust intrigued me by its integrated team practice approach where women are cared for by a group of known midwives and when she goes into labour all her care during labour/birth and in the postnatal period is provided by her known midwives within one environment.'

Hannah Wilson (2014) writing in a midwifery journal on how her elective shaped her is worth a read. Like Becky, she undertook an elective in a midwife-led unit which provided her with opportunities to observe holistic midwifery practice. The environment of 'normality' further developed her thinking around the type of midwife she wanted to become (an expert in normal birth), and the pathways she should follow to be confident with women's ability to birth physiologically.

Becky sums up her experience:

'I was able to ascertain that the role of the midwife is essentially the same everywhere. Different Trusts enable midwives to practice in different ways depending on ethos, culture and local policies. Despite meeting women from various backgrounds and parity from differing regional areas, questions for midwives were similar, which highlighted the importance of being aware of the basic needs of women and individualizing care depending on what is relevant for each woman's situation. My experience also reignited my belief that normal birth does happen and that women centred care is of the highest priority. Taking care back to basics, and loving the woman no matter who she is and where she has come from. Being compassionate towards her and her family, helping her oxytocin to flow. I have also begun to learn how to be mindful. Taking note of the woman's wishes for her birth, setting the right environment for her and reflecting on my own attitudes towards pregnancy and birth, ensuring this doesn't affect the care I give to a woman. In my journey of mindfulness I also realize that taking time for myself is important. Long shifts are demanding both physically and emotionally, on oneself and the family.'

Once you have decided on where you would like to be placed, you will need to write well in advance to the nominated education link within the Trust, continuing all the while to liaise with the relevant University staff. This is to ensure your request can be accommodated including providing you with appropriate mentoring. Remember that students from other universities may well be seeking these same opportunities, so there may be some competition for placements. Midwifery lecturers who link to the various clinical sites will be able to help you with names of contacts and email addresses if necessary. The placement team and your PT/AA will request confirmation of your plans at least 6 months before your elective begins. One of the advantages to the 'staycation with a twist' is that it enables you to have hands-on experience, as the clinical sites already have your University's students on placement there and contracts are in place. You might also get to do shifts with members of your cohort who are normally placed in that area; they will be friendly faces and will show you the ropes!

UK based but outside the locality of your University placements

Undertaking this option enables you to experience care anywhere within the United Kingdom where students from your University are not normally based. However, this opportunity will usually be 'observation status only' unless your University has a formal placement agreement with the NHS Trust you are seeking to gain experience in. Observer status means you will not be allowed to initiate or participate in the care or treatment of pregnant women and is typically time limited.

You will always be under the supervision of a registered practitioner. In some instances, you may be able to obtain an 'honorary contract' from the hospital where you are seeking to be placed, which would enable you to have an element of hands-on experience.

You will need to write to the Head of Midwifery (HOM) or identified midwifery education link for that Trust to obtain the necessary agreements. This again should be done well in advance to gain confirmation of your attendance and ensure you will be mentored by a registered midwife. Often, prior to accepting you in a placement outside the locality of your University, the HOM or the educational lead from the particular NHS Trust will request a letter from your PT/AA stating you are of good character and a genuine student attending your University. In addition, disclosure and barring service (DBS) clearance checks will need confirming. This is a screening process which flags up any previous criminal cautions or convictions, an essential requirement for professions which involve contact with vulnerable members of the public. A number of other conditions may be applicable such as the following:

- A copy of your intended learning outcomes.

- Evidence of manual handling and basic life support training.

- Evidence of occupational health clearance including immunisation screening.

- Completion of University elective information documents.

What do you need to consider if going elsewhere in the United Kingdom?

■ Finance – you will need to cover travelling and accommodation costs yourself.

■ Family commitments.

■ The demands of your course, can you manage the time?

Overseas elective

This option enables you to gain experience of midwifery care anywhere in the world and is often chosen by students who have family and friends abroad, or those seeking to pursue midwifery careers in other countries. Mostly, however, students choose this option because they would like to observe midwifery practice in another country. An important condition to be aware of is that you cannot gain hands-on experience unless you have the appropriate indemnity cover. Without this cover, which is a form of insurance which protects 'patients from harm', the placement is observational only and may again be time limited. Some universities allow you to add on your annual leave to extend your stay (Fig. 8.1).

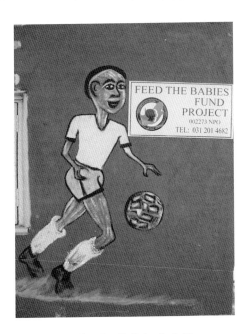

Figure 8.1 Feed the Babies Fund: a charity based in Durban, South Africa.

The advantages of an overseas elective

■ Experience healthcare within global settings where resources may not be as plentiful as within the United Kingdom and observe challenging/different working practices (see Vignette 8.2).

■ Experience working across multicultural settings which increases your awareness of cultural differences.

■ Improve your communication skills by working with women and their families where English is not their language.

■ Opportunity to utilise competencies acquired during your midwifery programme, for example teaching students or midwives in that country (see Vignette 8.2).

■ Compare and contrast models of midwifery care (see extracts of Becky Fry's experience).

Vignette 8.2   Laura's elective in Hoima, Uganda

Having heard about two students' overseas elective placements to Uganda towards the end of my first year, their passion and accounts of experiences fuelled my enthusiasm to visit Uganda in my own elective placement. During 22 June–8 July 2013, I had the complete privilege to travel to and work across two sites in Uganda: Hoima Regional Referral Hospital and Azur Christian clinic.

A small group of us met with two midwives who had previously spent time in Uganda working on a number of occasions. Flights and accommodation were booked and the rough total for the 2-week trip was £1500. The accommodation we stayed in provided all we required and comprised of twin rooms with a bathroom where, if you were lucky, you'd have a lovely warm shower! Prior to entering Uganda, we had to be immunised against yellow fever (at the cost of £65!!) and immunisation against hepatitis A was also recommended. Antimalarial tablets were also another extortionate cost but obviously entirely necessary for the duration of our stay. All of us were completely willing to self-fund; however, we did apply to the BU Global Horizons fund and I was awarded £800 to help towards costs. We set up a group 'justgiving' page where we managed to raise approximately £1500 through donations from friends and family along with an array of knitted items for newborns and toys/sweets for the children we visited at the Mustard Seed Orphanage. This money was raised primarily in order to purchase teaching aids for the School of Midwifery and equipment to be used in Hoima and Azur hospitals. All of the delivery and suture packs, swabs etc. we used whilst working there were obtained from local UK Trusts which would otherwise have disposed of them.

Intercultural skills in today's society are critical in effective communication; the acknowledgement of differences in culture, views and expectations will aid this. Through going to Uganda, I have expanded these skills by working collaboratively with midwives who looked after women from a variety of cultures, practising in difficult and very different circumstances from those that I am used to.

Whilst in Uganda, I was able to practice raw skills of midwifery. With many women coming in labouring, or in the antenatal period for various reasons having received very little or no antenatal care, key skills such as simply listening to women as well as abdominal palpations and the use of Pinard stethoscopes were of paramount importance. The development of my non-verbal communication skills will help me to support and interact with women worldwide, irrespective of cultural beliefs; it truly is surprising how much information can be conveyed when neither party speaks a word of the other's language!

Dealing with the 'high-risk' African population meant it was necessary to utilise skills surrounding the management of obstetric emergencies. I was also involved in the teaching of these to six Ugandan student midwives, empowering them with knowledge whilst learning from them too. Although management is dependent on resources, and therefore slightly different in Uganda, the principles of controlling a PPH, for example, remain the same. Reacting to these situations and knowing what to do for real has helped me to build my own confidence in practice. Similarly, undertaking and teaching neonatal resuscitation has enabled me to consolidate practice further.

Although nothing can ever prepare you for maternal and neonatal morbidity or mortality, experiencing it in this situation has equipped me with invaluable skills. Witnessing how grief affects people in very different ways and learning from both UK and Ugandan midwives how to support women and their families during this time can be directly transferable to my role as a newly qualified midwife.

On the whole, in both Hoima and Azur women received very little postnatal care. I feel this is primarily due to the business of the unit as well as there often being a lack of staff. In Azur, I helped to create a basic double-sided postnatal proforma, one side for mother and the other baby, to be utilised on a postnatal ward round. It included space to document basic observations and informed staff of what is considered as 'normal ranges' as well as key words (e.g. breasts, lochia and perineum for mother and skin, cord and eyes for baby) as prompts for midwives/student midwives to base their postnatal assessment upon. The aim was to provide the staff with documentation of continued postnatal care, highlighting some factors (particularly sepsis) that necessitate referrals to the obstetric/paediatric team.

However, it wasn't all work . . . We had two nights staying at Paraa Safari Lodge, which was absolute luxury! We went on two sunrise safaris and one sunset safari where saw everything from giraffes to hyenas, elephants to warthogs, a leopard up a tree and even a three-legged lion! This was then followed by a drink or two at the pool bar, far too much food and a swim/sunbathe in the African sun. We also spent many evenings at the local orphanage playing ball games, pushing swings, giving out Haribo sweets or just having a cuddle with the little ones.

We were so well supported by the midwives whom we went out there with; daily debriefings took place where we were able to discuss scenarios we saw,

(continued)

were involved in and things we wanted to achieve – often with local Ugandan gin to help!

Before going on this placement, I had to maintain the mentality that I was not going to change the world, but my aim was to make a difference to the individual women and their babies that I had the privilege of caring for. I hope I achieved this; two short weeks truly highlighted how precious life is. I had such an incredible and steep learning curve and have absolute admiration for the midwives and women who make the best of their situation, yet still wear the biggest smile. How very lucky we are to have the National Health Service with open access to healthcare, no matter who we are, what we need or how much money we have. Uganda has completely stolen my heart and I can't wait to go back as a qualified midwife!

Laura Briers
Previous student, Bournemouth University
Reproduced with permission of Laura Briers

■ An international activity enhances your curriculum vitae (CV) and your own personal skills.

Practicalities to consider

■ Are you fit and well? If you have a chronic condition which requires regular prescribed medication, make sure you have enough medication to take with you including copies of your prescription, so that if you run out or lose your luggage you will be able to obtain more (Stanley 2014). It may be prudent to keep these items in your hand luggage. If necessary, speak to your general practitioner (GP) before you book your elective (Plymouth University 2012).

■ Know your emergency contact numbers and keep them handy. You probably won't ever need to use them but if you do make sure they are easily found (Plymouth University 2012).

■ Weather in some countries can be extreme, depending on the time of year.

For instance, it can be very hot during the day and really cold at night. Ensure your clothing copes with both extremes. Remember to pack your sunscreen as well.

■ Pack a first aid kit. Travel pocket kits start at around £10.00 from an online retailer such as http://www.nomadtravel.co.uk/c/204/Travel-Store. You could just make one up yourself, packing items such as plasters, dressings and antiseptic creams in a waterproof bag. Remember all liquid items if carried in your hand luggage should be under 100 mL.

■ Meet up with people who have been to the country/institution you intend to visit (Stanley 2014). Laura was able to meet up with midwives who had previously been out to Uganda. If you are able to meet up with people before you go, it may help with your planning, such as logistics (travelling to/from airport, accommodation, cultural issues) and any other issues you may not have considered.

■ Your University may also require you to undertake a risk assessment exercise on the placement you are attending. Ensure all paperwork is completed and sent to the relevant departments.

Start planning for your elective at least a year in advance. Usually in the second year of your programme, lecturers will introduce the concept of an international elective. You will be required to fill in numerous forms and speak with lecturers/international practice placement coordinators culminating in you organising and managing your whole trip. The sooner the better, as once you've made up your mind you can begin to consider sources of funding to sponsor your trip and the practicalities of your chosen destination. If you find it altogether too much, established companies such as Work the World have tailor-made electives and placements and in accordance with your aims/objectives will organise everything for you.

Think about where you would like to go based on the type of experience you are seeking. This will influence your choice of country/healthcare setting. Lisa Common (2007), who was a student at Nottingham University, organised an elective in Zambia, because she wanted a placement in a rural area where midwives relied solely on their midwifery skills. Just from preparing for her trip, Lisa's world changed in many positive ways. Her skills in planning and organisation were increased and this impacted on her overall confidence. Ultimately, however, her elective provided her with purpose and aspirations. Lisa wanted to positively influence change for women in resource-poor countries where women's healthcare needs are not always top priority. One of the priorities for third-year BU students Jo Lake and Zoe Shama on their elective in Rwanda was to spend time at the Kabgayi School of Nursing and Midwifery in Gitarama to observe any differences between midwifery training in Rwanda and the United Kingdom (Fig. 8.2). Here is part of what they discovered:

'It turns out that in principle there isn't much difference between the 2 courses. In Rwanda the midwifery course is a 3 year diploma and the students spend half of their time in theory blocks and half in clinical practice which is very similar to the UK. Their 1st placement is in the community setting which again is the same as the UK. However, their community placements are somewhat different to ours because they do antenatal visits with a community health worker (instead of a midwife) whose role is essentially to assess the mothers' situation e.g. living situation/conditions and other family members/dependents and to discuss nutrition, hygiene and where to go/who to see during the pregnancy. Domitilla described these placements as essential for students to gain an understanding of the contexts in which women are having babies. Many of the women are poor, have little income and a small home. They may already be undernourished, anaemic or have an underlying medical condition or infection that they are unaware of so the advice they are given early on is vital. Other placements for the students includes health centres (similar to Midwifery-Led Units in the UK) and district hospitals (like Obstetric-Led Units) and sometimes they also go to a big

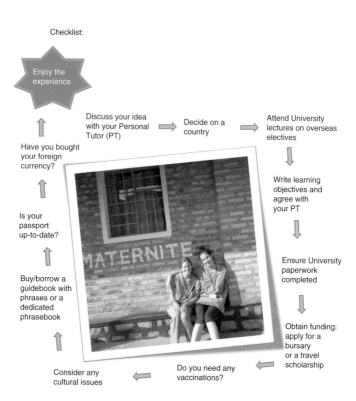

Checklist:

Enjoy the experience

Discuss your idea with your Personal Tutor (PT)

Decide on a country

Attend University lectures on overseas electives

Have you bought your foreign currency?

Write learning objectives and agree with your PT

Is your passport up-to-date?

Ensure University paperwork completed

Buy/borrow a guidebook with phrases or a dedicated phrasebook

Obtain funding: apply for a bursary or a travel scholarship

Consider any cultural issues

Do you need any vaccinations?

Figure 8.2 Checklist for electives. Two third-year Bournemouth University midwifery students on their elective in Rwanda.

centralised hospital of which there are 4 in Rwanda; 3 in Kigali and 1 in Butare. Students are not permitted to facilitate births until their second year, supposedly only needing to "catch" 10 babies throughout their training (we say supposedly because further research implies that this number does not match up with what the United Nations Population Fund report suggests). As we'll explain later these numbers could easily be achieved in a district hospital within a couple of days! Students also have objectives to achieve during each placement enabling them to become competent in all areas of midwifery care ready for qualification. One difference here is that student midwives must do a national exam and will not receive their midwifery registration if they don't pass.'

Many universities already have strong educational links in particular countries and making use of these contacts will make life a lot smoother for you. Another option is to join an association which has already forged partnerships and an ongoing commitment to address the needs identified by the people of that country. The members of these associations (variety of healthcare and non-healthcare practitioners) regularly visit to provide training and any other service thought necessary by the local people. The advantages of joining one of these schemes are that you will be able to undertake some practice under the guidance of registered practitioners. Laura Briers, a previous BU midwifery student, joined the Basingstoke Hoima Partnership for Health for her election in Hoima, Uganda (http://www.hampshirehospitals.nhs.uk/about-us/global-health-links.aspx). Her vignette reflects the joys and tribulations of her experience.

Planning your expenses

As can be seen from Laura's vignette, expenses for a trip overseas can be considerable. It is, however, vitally important you consider and plan how much your elective is likely to cost because if you are intending to apply for funding/sponsorship either for an overseas elective or for a 'staycation with a twist', knowing your expenses can make a difference between a successful and an unsuccessful application. The Iolanthe Trust, which has many more applications for funding than they can afford to sponsor, suggest an application which has no specific details on costs (just a lump sum being identified) or excessive costs is unlikely to be successful (Fig. 8.3). They offer detailed guidance on completing applications for their *own* student awards; however, the advice is likely to be applicable to other sources of funding you may be considering. Funding bodies either offer a fixed amount or will provide funding based on the needs of your application.

Where can I get funding for an elective placement?

■ Your own University may have sources of funding that you will need to apply for. In addition, the Student Union (SU) based at your institution may either fund you or direct you to funding opportunities.

■ Plan a fund raising event: i.e. cake sale, sponsored bike ride, sponsored run/swim; the list is endless.

■ Some students have used 'crowdfunding' sites to raise funds for their elective.

■ Charities such as the following:

– **Iolanthe Trust Awards** (http://www.iolanthe.org/): Usually open for applications around November each year and closes the following January. There is guidance available on the website if you are considering applying for an award from them.

– **Wellbeing of Women** (http://www.wellbeingofwomen.org.uk/): Elective bursaries open for applications in March of each year. Medical students

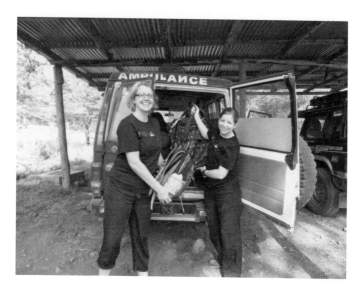

Figure 8.3 Two third-year Bournemouth University midwifery students on their elective in Kenya.

are also able to apply for these bursaries. Applications can be for electives both within the United Kingdom and overseas.

– **Royal College of Midwives** (RCM; https://www.rcm.org.uk/): Annual Midwifery Awards – open to all members of the RCM.

– **Money4MedStudents** (http://www .money4medstudents.org/budgeting-for-your-elective): Provides practical, unbiased information and advice on sources of funding.

■ Money for Christmas and birthdays.

■ Some midwifery journals pay for articles; consider writing about your elective plans like Lisa did (Common 2007). She also won an essay writing

competition which had a cash prize and applied and was successfully chosen as a contestant on The Weakest Link.

■ Selling items on eBay. Your 'junk' is someone else's joy!

■ Car boot sales if you have time and energy. Again it's amazing what people will buy (Common 2007).

What sort of questions might you see on an application for funding form?

■ Your personal details, such as name, date of birth, contact address, email address and telephone numbers.

■ Details of your educational institution.

■ Dates of when you started midwifery course and proposed date of completion.

■ Name of your Personal Tutor or Academic Advisor and their contact details.

■ Your CV. It is important to keep this updated on a regular basis and stored electronically as it will be needed for when you apply for jobs (see Chapter 9).

■ Reasons for the request (this can be an elective placement, attendance at a study day or conference or undertaking a course, i.e. baby massage).

■ Dates of proposed elective.

■ Location of elective (contact institution or contact you are visiting).

■ Whether your elective has been confirmed or you are awaiting confirmation.

■ Full costs (travel, accommodation, fees etc.).

■ Any additional attempts to raise money for your elective including applications to other funding bodies.

■ Additional information to support your application (word allowance usually limited, e.g. 100 words).

All applications should be completed electronically; you should avoid handwritten forms. Ensure you have completed each section appropriately and include any relevant documents requested by the funding body, e.g. a supporting statement from your PT indicating approval for your plans and from your contact at the placement.

(Adapted from The Iolanthe Midwifery Trust application for Iolanthe Student Awards, 2014 and Gulsin & Johnston 2011.)

Budget planner

Begin by listing all your expenses: an example is shown in Table 8.1, where a student was considering an elective in Haiti.

The estimated total for a Haiti elective (without extras) amounts to around £1500.00. The overall costs do not take into account spending money, and whether you will undertake any sightseeing. This is a large outlay for a student; however, the benefits you will obtain from the placement probably outweigh the negatives such as expenses. Laura's concluding words demonstrate how much her elective meant to her:

> 'I had such an incredible and steep learning curve and have absolute admiration for the midwives and women in Uganda who make the best of their situation, yet still wear the biggest smile. How very lucky we are to have the National Health Service with open access to healthcare, no matter who we are, what we need or how much money we have. Uganda has completely stolen my heart and I can't wait to go back as a qualified midwife!'

Erasmus Programme

An alternative option for an elective is a scheme called the Erasmus Programme (http://www.erasmus.ac.uk/), which is a European network of universities that have partnered together to enable student mobility across European institutions. If your University belongs to this

Table 8.1 Example of a budget planner.

Item	Cost	Notes
1. Travel: return flights to country of choice Haiti: Port-au-Prince	£800.00	
2. Transfer between airports	£600.00	Costs include accommodation, food and cost of a translator. Do not include costing for travel to and from UK airport
3. Travel insurance	£20.00	
4. Immunisations: recommended for Haiti		Malarone strongly advised: 1 tablet = £2.50 23 tablets = £58.00
Yellow fever	£45.00	
Anti-malarial tablets:	20 tablets:	
Chloroquine	£2.50	
Malarone	£58.00	
Hepatitis B	£45.00	
Diphtheria	£30.00	Combined with tetanus and polio
5. Accommodation for 2–3 weeks		See above
6. Living expenses: Food Personal		See above
7. Other		

Adapted from Gulsin and Johnston (2011).

scheme, you will be able to undertake an elective within the European Union. Bournemouth University, for example, has joined the Erasmus Socrates exchange programme and midwifery students are able to undertake an elective in one of three countries: Sweden, Denmark and Finland. The benefit of belonging to this exchange programme is that midwifery students are able to undertake practice for 12 weeks in a hospital affiliated to the University and be officially mentored by midwives when in practice. Your practice hours can usually be accredited against your required hours but you will have to produce evidence to show you have worked them. In some cases, you may be able to undertake an aspect of theory whilst in the host University, and you will gain credits for any learning but you will not be able to use these credits to prop up your undergraduate degree.

Benefits of an Erasmus placement

The benefits are similar to an overseas placement:

- Broadens your knowledge and awareness of healthcare outside your normal country.

- Opportunities to learn about different models of healthcare.

- Raises your awareness of multicultural issues both within society and in healthcare institutions.

- Prepares you for the potential to work in other countries.

- Make new friends and experience a new country.

- Learn a new language, eat different food.

- Good for your CV by enhancing your employability and career prospects.

Other benefits

- The EU sponsors Erasmus placements.

- You receive a grant for the duration of your overseas elective (currently it is around €370 per month; however, rates do vary each academic year).

- Because partnerships are already established, your University is able to organise the placement directly.

- English is widely spoken (you should still learn some basic words from the country) and students from the United Kingdom are generally well received.

Criteria for an Erasmus placement

- Places are limited. If you are interested, you need to apply in the spring term of your second year to undertake your placement the following semester (usually October of the following academic year).

- Placements must be for a minimum of 3 months.

- Placements can only take place where your University has a current Erasmus mobility agreement.

- You must be of an EU nationality.

- Your Erasmus grant helps towards your living costs, which enables you to study and work at a partner University. This grant is issued in addition to all other grants, bursaries or loans you may already be receiving.

Practicalities

- The demands of your University course and meeting completion dates for skills, competencies, EU numbers and clinical hours.

- Funding – sponsorship versus self-financing.

- Any commitments you already have at home.

- Practical organisation, such as organising or renewing passports, and obtaining visas (although not usually required within the EU) and travel insurance, can all be time-consuming activities.

- Language and how you will communicate, although many countries within the EU are fluent in English.

Catherine Ricklesford, a previous student from Bournemouth University, has published an article on her Erasmus

Socrates placement at the Karolinska Institutet (KI) in Stockholm, Sweden. She thoroughly enjoyed her experience and found it extremely beneficial. To read more of her story, it can be found at the following link: http://www.wellbeingofwomen.org.uk/downloads/file/02_research/pdf/2007%202008%20Elective%20Reports/Ricklesford%20Report.pdf.

Other ideas/opportunities during your elective

Investigate a research career

If you are interested in research, there may be an opportunity for you to spend time with a midwifery researcher to consider whether this may be a future career option for you. Midwifery researchers have a wide and varied role and choosing to spend part of your elective with him/her will reveal some of the following aspects of their job:

- Clinical research in practice.

- Working with service users.

- Research governance.

- Funding opportunities.

- Grant applications.

- Report writing.

- Writing for publication.

- Conference presentation.

Career profile of Research Midwife is available at http://www.rcm.org.uk/college/your-career/students/student-life-e-newsletter/student-life-october-2010/career-profile-research-midwife/.

Independent midwifery

Experiencing midwifery care outside the NHS can be another option for you to pursue. Independent midwives (IMs) are self-employed and work independently of the NHS, although some will do bank shifts within their local Trusts. As with many of the other options already explored in this chapter, you will need to contact the organisation Independent Midwives UK (IMUK) in good time either to arrange for work experience or to shadow an IM. As with electives arranged outside the locality of your University or placements overseas, it will be observation only unless you can secure professional indemnity insurance. IMUK also provide workshops which focus on developing entrepreneurial skills and advice on setting up independent practice.

Shadowing and work experience advice is available at http://www.independentmidwives.org.uk/?node=12910.

Midwifery services via social enterprises

1 **One to One**: It is a service which has been commissioned by the NHS and provides maternity care in partnership with women and midwives within local communities. Their philosophy is focused on birth as a normal event and promotes home birth as a choice for all women who are considered low-risk. Placements are offered to midwifery students.

For further information, access the following link: http://www.onetoonemidwives.org/.

2 Neighbourhood Midwives: It is similar to One to One but was devised and implemented by midwives. Neighbourhood Midwives are known as a social enterprise business where any surplus made by the 'company' is put back into the business to achieve their social aims. Limited places are available for student elective placements as demand is high. Contact your local Neighbourhood Midwives as soon as you can although there may already be a waiting list.

For further information, access the following link: http://www.neighbourhoodmidwives.org.uk/index.php.

What next following your elective?

■ Reflect and revisit original learning outcomes. Were they achieved and if not, is there anything you can do to rectify the situation?

■ Are you able to share your experience? Some universities provide sessions on your final University day and others may facilitate student theme days where you may be able to 'showcase' your story.

■ Are you able to disseminate at your local hospital? If like Laura you joined an established association, it is good practice to feedback on your experience.

■ Consider an article for the RCM or other midwifery journals. Successful funding applications require a publication or two following your elective experience.

■ Submit a paper for a conference (such as the RCM Annual Conference or Student Midwives' Conference).

■ Is it possible that you can maintain a relationship with the community you visited? Perhaps one of your intended learning outcomes would have been to make the contact sustainable (Einterz 2008). Has this been achieved? If not, are you able to suggest ways in which contacts can be sustained?

■ There may be more formal expectations post elective from some universities to produce a written reflective report. Plymouth University encourage students to submit an account of their elective to include planning and undertaking the elective based on the following sections:

– Initial aims and ideas.

– Discussion of objectives.

– Personal reflections on the experience.

– What you bring back.

– The elective host organisation.

– Country demographics.

– Public health issues.

– Foreign and Commonwealth Office/ Department of Health advice.

– Local health issues.

– Your personal health and safety issues (Plymouth University 2012).

Once you have written your report, consider publication. Speak with your PT/AA who will help you get the report ready for publication in a relevant journal. It's great seeing your name in print.

Conclusion

Generally electives do not benefit from lastminute.com type of arrangements. The advantages gained will be outweighed by stresses and strains of not being prepared and important learning may be lost. Start planning and negotiations early on, even as early as your first year. A recent trawl on an Internet-based web chatline dedicated to student midwives revealed that first-year students were already thinking about their electives and possible sources of funding. Others hadn't started their midwifery course and were excited at the prospect of going to a foreign country to experience midwifery during their training. The majority of students, however, were just going to stay 'at home' and spend time in midwife-led units or with Independent Midwives.

Travelling abroad has its risks (Stanley 2014); situations in some overseas countries change overnight and what was once a safe and secure country when you started with your arrangements may turn out to be extremely unstable when the time comes for you to travel. The Foreign and Commonwealth Office (FCO; https://www.gov.uk/foreign-travel-advice) offers useful travel advice around safety and security, including advising you on local customs and law. For example, when travelling to Rwanda photography of government buildings is prohibited and plastic bags have been banned for environmental reasons. Always check with the FCO for up-to-date travel advice. Also, circumstances may change whilst you are in a particular country, i.e. a coup where the sitting government has been overthrown by its army, or there's a natural disaster. If you are in need of help, it will be your responsibility to contact the British Embassy, the Consulate or High Commissioner for advice and support (Stanley 2014).

When travelling overseas, it is important to remember you are a guest in that country; always respect the cultures and beliefs of the community you are visiting, even if these are challenging to you (British Medical Association 2009). Undertake research on customs and codes of the particular country before you leave, for example dress codes are important in some countries and you may offend local people if you are inappropriately dressed. Gender roles may be vastly different from what you are used to: in some cultures men will make treatment decisions for women; in other words, women themselves do not make decisions about their own healthcare. Remain culturally aware by being open and sensitive to these differences and try not to be critical (British Medical Association 2009). Learn simple phrases; saying hello in the local language or even learning basic sentences such as "how much" will show the locals you have tried to learn a little about their language and are trying to communicate with them (Anderson 2013). They will respect your efforts, so don't be embarrassed to try out the phrases you have learnt.

There are many benefits to undertaking an elective whether locally, nationally or internationally; therefore, plan early and be proactive. See Box 8.1 for top tips from Bournemouth University students. Take advantage of any help on offer; make good use of reliable contacts, and most of all enjoy the experience. Remember you are an ambassador for the country where you are undertaking your midwifery training and for your University. I leave you with the following quote:

'. . . you must apply the highest standards that the course has prepared you for. In particular we draw your attention to the issue of consent. This is especially important if you are working with clients or patients but also if you are working in any environment where it is necessary to engage with other people.'

(Plymouth University 2012)

Box 8.1 Top Tips

■ Photocopy all important documents and take with you (passport, visa, insurance details, credit card (CC) details and contact details of CC company, or take a photo of your passport/relevant documents and keep stored on your phone/tablet as a jpeg).

■ Start preparing early for electives – destination of choice and consider sources of funding.

■ Try and travel in pairs for support.

■ Apply for funding well in advance. I managed to get my flight paid for by a very small charity supporting education I found on the Internet.

■ Consider your weaknesses, areas you're not confident in where you can place yourself on elective.

■ Get the most out of your elective, no matter where you spend it.

■ Go somewhere different for your elective, local hospitals and abroad (if possible).

■ Sweden (Erasmus Placement) was amazing.

■ Phone chosen hospital before writing to ask to work there as the HOM is often not the person to talk to.

■ *Definitely* go to another hospital within the locality of your University.

■ Try to work in areas you are less confident in during your elective (to try and conquer your fears).

■ On your elective use your time to go to places that really interest you as they really affect your placement experience.

Midwifery students from Bournemouth University

References

Anderson A (2013) Backpacking Diplomacy. Available at http://www.backpackingdiplomacy.com/respecting-culture-when-you-travel/ (last accessed 21 July 2014).

British Medical Association (2009) Ethics and medical electives in resource-poor countries. A tool kit. Available at http://bma.org.uk (last accessed 21 July 2014).

Common L (2007) Organising an elective placement in Zambia. *Midwifery Matters* 114: 16–17.

Einterz EM (2008) The medical student elective in Africa: advice from the field. *CMAJ* 178: 1461–1463.

Gulsin GS, Johnston PW (2011) Funding your elective. Ten steps to bring you closer to your destination. *Student BMJ* 19: d5851.

Plymouth University (2012) Overseas Electives Handbook. Available at http://www1.plymouth.ac.uk/placements/poppi/newhealth/Documents/Overseas%20elective%20handbook%202012-2013.pdf (last accessed 21 July 2014).

Stanley D (2014) How to prepare for an international elective clinical placement. Available at http://www.midirs.org/how-to-prepare-for-an-international-elective-clinical-placement/ (last accessed 21 July 2014).

Way S, Little C (2014) Elective Placement Midwifery Students. PowerPoint presentation, Bournemouth University.

Wilson H (2014) An education in midwifery: the role of an elective placement in shaping a student's approach. *Br J Midwifery* 22: 35–41.

Further resources

Emma Barton & Amanda Gill, third-year midwifery students at Bournemouth University, undertook an elective in Sweden. See their story at the following link: https://www.youtube.com/watch?v=Ks7XjQld4xs.

Work the World: Tailor-made placements in Africa, Asia & South America (worktheworld.co.uk).

Overseas midwifery placements – planning your elective (http://www.rcm.org.uk/college/your-career/students/student-life-e-newsletter/student-life-march-2012/overseas-midwifery-placements-planning-your-elective/#sthash.4cuaRYvy.dpuf).

The Electives Network: http://www.electives.net/.

Midwives for Haiti: http://www.midwivesforhaiti.org/.

The Iolanthe Midwifery Trust: Applying for an award (http://www.iolanthe.org/Applying_for_an_Award.cfm).

White Ribbon Alliance for Safe Motherhood (WRA): www.whiteribbonalliance.org.

Chapter 9
WHAT NEXT?

Faye Doris

Introduction

You are now at an exciting point of your midwifery programme and would have been taking increasing responsibility as a student midwife during the final year of your programme. You are also aware of the knowledge, skills and experience that you have gained and the confidence you have in providing care for women and babies when the parameters are normal. Application of theory to practice, being 'with woman' and providing safe, evidenced-based care is a mantra and many of you would have developed your own philosophies based on this. Experience would also have been gained in recognising and caring for mothers and babies with the common high-risk conditions such as caring for a woman with a hypertensive disorder or being involved in the management of a shoulder dystocia during labour or a post-partum haemorrhage. You are therefore likely to be thinking of your first midwifery post. This chapter considers the next stages of your journey. It will discuss preparing for interviews, the ongoing professional requirements, regulation and guidance that will provide the framework for your future practice. Where references are made to particular resources, useful websites will be provided at the end of this chapter. The aim is to provide you with some of the tools and evidence to assist your transition to being a newly qualified midwife and continuing to learn as a practitioner of midwifery.

Preparing for interviews

Preparing for an interview is very similar to planning an essay. It involves many stages and requires you to pay attention to detail. It is more than applying for a job, for the better prepared you are, the more confident you will feel and the more likely you are to make a good impression and get that job. Although you may believe that your main aim is to be employed, a successful interview would require more than this. Start by relooking at the job description and your application. Where did you apply for a job?

The Hands-on Guide to Midwifery Placements, First Edition.
Edited by Luisa Cescutti-Butler and Margaret Fisher.
© 2016 John Wiley & Sons, Ltd. Published 2016 by John Wiley & Sons, Ltd.

Are you staying in the same unit?

You may choose to apply for your first post in the unit where you are currently doing your midwifery course and where you feel you know everyone, like the culture and are familiar with the philosophy of care. You have been shortlisted for an interview and you are confident because you are well known as one of 'their students'. This is a false sense of security, for all job interviews follow a stringent process and are competitive. You have an advantage in that you are familiar with the culture, policies and model of care. Have you looked objectively at the Trust or unit's external website recently? What does it tell you about the Trust or unit? Are there any surprises? What do users of the service say about the care that they received and the staff that cared for them? How have they evaluated the service? You will be able to gather this information from a number of sources. You may ask a mother or father/partner directly, you may get some information from the Department of Health in the United Kingdom Friends and Family Test, the Care Quality Commission's (CQC) User Survey or a Care Quality Commission's Report for that Trust. This would provide a wide source of information and a rich background to inform your interview discussion, presentation or response to questions. It may also direct you to a question that you may wish to ask. In this scenario, do not make assumptions of whom you know or what you know. Prepare as if you are considering this unit totally new and in a similar way as if you were moving on to another.

Are you moving away?

The principles discussed above are the same if you are applying to a different Trust. The key factor here is why you chose this specific unit. It could be nearer home or moving away. It may be a different type of experience or model of care. So ask yourself:

■ What do you know about the Trust or unit, its philosophy of care, number of births per year and intervention rate?

■ Is the population of women more diverse or complex than you have been accustomed to?

■ Does it offer particular experiences such as a cardiac specialist unit for mother or baby?

Having read the previous section, you would now anticipate gathering information about the Trust from their website, women, fathers/partners, midwives and students who have experienced that unit. Have you undertaken an informal visit, arranged this prior to the interview or spoken to a senior staff member from the unit? A practice development midwife is a useful person to contact, for they are able to provide broad information and comment on the learning available to staff within the Trust.

Victoria Fields, a preceptee midwife, shares her experiences of getting ready to be interviewed for her first midwifery post in Vignette 9.1.

Vignette 9.1   Preparing for interviews

'Interviews can be a particularly nerve racking time; at the time of my first interview I felt like the last 3 years of my life were hanging on a knife edge and everything I had learnt, all the exams I had passed and essays I had written had come down to a 1 hour window in my life. This is, of course, not the case. A good interviewer will listen to what you are saying and give you plenty of chances to impress them. Do not be afraid of the interview; it is not a process of interrogation, it is a fantastic opportunity to showcase the skills and knowledge you have learnt and is a chance to sell yourself as a professional. Be proud of ALL your achievements, however small. It is normal to have pre-interview nerves. It is important to remember that they have already selected you from a plethora of applicants; they already like what you have got to offer.

It is important you are confident with emergency scenarios and CTG interpretations, as these are now seen as essential key skills to demonstrate at interview. They came up in every pre- and post-registration interview I have done, in some cases before I was even invited to a face-to-face interview.

Some key points to remember are to thoroughly research the hospital. Be aware of the answers to common questions such as why do you want to work at this hospital, why this area and even why midwifery?

I have found that quoting research not only is an effective way of demonstrating your practice is relevant and up to date, but also shows the interviewer you have prepared for the interview and are aware of important current midwifery issues.

Finally, remember that lifelong learning and development is an important part of midwifery. Including career goals for the future in your personal statement and at interview shows that you are thinking ahead. Showing eagerness for progression is an asset to your future employer and yourself.'

Victoria Fields
Preceptee midwife and previous Plymouth University student
Reproduced with permission of Victoria Fields

Curriculum vitae

It is likely that you would have prepared a curriculum vitae (CV) as part of your application or are planning to send one with an application that you are about to make, so let us consider what a good CV may look like. Firstly, consider what a curriculum vitae is. It is a document that provides additional information to support an application form for a job. It tells a prospective employer something about you but more importantly tells the reader where you have come from, what you have achieved and where you want to go. A literature search will find many books or journal articles on the subject. You will also find useful websites such as *The Guardian* newspaper in the United Kingdom (see address at the end of the chapter) providing guidance on writing a good curriculum vitae. Whilst these are all helpful, you will find that every time you apply for a job you need to think of the audience who will be reading this information and tailor your CV to suit them, the job description and the person specification of the post for which you are applying. This is so even when you are applying for the same type of job, for example a newly qualified midwife's position. You will therefore need to review your CV for every individual post to see that it demonstrates the qualities, qualifications, skills and experience required. When preparing for an interview as a final year student midwife you will be commenting on the qualifications that you have to date but giving some indication of the progress on your programme. This may be that 'I have successfully completed all assessments to date.'

Format of CV

The usual length of a CV is two sides of an A4 page. See Box 9.1 for example. This has been adapted from the Royal College of Midwives of the United Kingdom i-folio website (http://www.ilearn.rcm.org.uk/).

The above is a very basic curriculum vitae outline which you could build on during your professional career. If you have a format that you already use, review it as suggested earlier to fit the job for which you are applying.

Pitfalls with CVs

Avoid the following common mistakes in what is a professional document:

- jargon
- abbreviations
- grammatical errors
- spelling errors
- repetition

Think of the comments that you received on your written work as a student; they also apply to your CV. Read your work aloud and get someone else to check it for errors. Do not exaggerate your achievements that you cannot evidence at interview. Do not make negative comments such as 'I only achieved a pass degree or a 2:2.' It is the 'only' that is wrong in such a statement.

Presentation of your CV

This chapter started by saying that attention to detail was necessary when preparing for an interview. The previous statements have begun to illustrate some of this. Your CV should be presented as a professional document. It starts to say something about the standard of your record-keeping.

The typeface should be 12 font Arial or Times Roman. Look at your headings or text on each line. Do they start at the same point or are they erratic? Do you present them in a consistent manner? The Royal College of Midwives i-folio site, for those of you who have access to it, provides guidance about using tables in Microsoft Word to align your work and is well worth considering. You may have found another source that provides this information and this would also be useful. Avoid coloured font; black on pale yellow paper is known to be good practice.

Build on your CV throughout your career and you will find that it will look

Box 9.1 Sample curriculum vitae template

Name:

Address:

Email:

[Items below are no longer required in view of the Equality Act 2010]:
Date of Birth
Age
Sex
Marital Status
Religion

You may provide your telephone number at interview for making contact.

Profile: This is where you will sell yourself and say who you are. You must be able to evidence the statements made here at interview. You may choose to include in this section the headings from the Nursing and Midwifery Council (NMC)'s Essential Skills Clusters for midwifery headings with a sentence to indicate your achievements. These are 'Communication, Initial consultation between the woman and the midwife, Normal labour and birth, Initiation and continuance of breastfeeding and Medicines management' (NMC 2009).

Education:

Qualifications:

Other skills/achievements: This is where you would include whether you speak other languages, whether you can do sign language, voluntary work you have undertaken that demonstrates skills relevant to the job such as team working or leadership, awards or prizes at University, cohort representative, Peer Assisted Learning leader and so on. You must be able to evidence these or discuss them at an interview if asked.

References/referees: Referees need to be asked prior to submitting their names. It is better to say that referees can be supplied on request if you have not asked their permission as yet.

(Adapted from Royal College of Midwives (2014) i-folio website: http://www.ilearn.rcm.org.uk/.)

different based on your professional pathway and the type of evidence that you need to provide for a particular job. A clear example of this is the need for conferences, publications and research when applying for an academic post.

Personal statement

This usually forms part of any application form and is an important element that determines whether you are selected for an interview or not. When looked at in totality with the rest of the application and your curriculum vitae, it is important that you do not repeat yourself. Should your application form omit a section on personal statements, it is helpful to add this as an additional page to your curriculum vitae. Plan your statement and structure it. A SWOT (strengths, weaknesses, opportunities and threats) review of yourself in relation to the job applied for may be helpful in choosing the content of this statement. You must have in your structure a clear introduction, middle and conclusion or summary. Do not present a list of why you are ideally suited for the job. Think of what you would like to say as to why you would like to be considered for the job, then explain this.

Covering letter

Having done the preparation and completed your application and CV to a high standard, remember that if submitting this by post a formal covering letter will be required. The process is likely to be different for an online application, but always consider whether this will be needed. Apply the principles discussed above. You may want to prepare this, get someone to look at it for errors and keep it on file for future use. You would then review it to see if it remains relevant to each new application.

The actual interview

This section is presented as a list of good practice as you should now feel well prepared for your interview.

Things to do

■ Know where you are going, the place, room and time. Consult a map in advance.

■ Be punctual. Leave plenty of time to get there in case you get lost or encounter traffic problems.

■ Have available a contact name and number at the place of interview.

■ Have coins for the car park.

■ Dress professionally and remember clean shoes are also important.

■ A strong perfume or the smell of cigarette smoke on your clothes is distracting. Consider this in your dress for the day. Also remember that this may linger on your coat.

■ Have a copy of your job description and person specification, communication from the Human Resource (HR) Department of the Trust, your application form and CV with you. HR may ask you to bring specific documents with you such as your qualification certificates and others.

■ Turn your mobile off.

■ Remember to smile.

■ When being interviewed, do not fidget or be overfamiliar, particularly if you know the staff. Address them professionally, taking a cue from the way they speak to you. Do not assume that first names are the acceptable norm.

■ Consider some of the questions you may be asked having looked at the job description and person specifications. It is a bad idea to respond by saying 'I thought you would have asked me that.'

■ It is anticipated that you would have found out about shift times, rotation to wards, night and day duty in advance.

■ A thank you at the end is normal.

From the list above you will be clear about some of the things that you should and should not do at interview. Good luck.

Presentations

It is now becoming normal to ask you to do a presentation as part of your interview. Be prepared for this. Plan and structure it well, deconstruct the topic and answer the question asked. Read around the subject and complete a literature search as you prepare it. Some helpful guidance is presented below:

■ Use the medium that suits you best, such as PowerPoint or a poster. Is there another way of doing this, for example a storyboard? Do not be overambitious unless you are skilled in the medium you have chosen.

■ If you are planning to use PowerPoint, identify in advance whether a computer or projector is available.

■ Consider handouts; identify the number in your audience so that you can prepare enough.

■ Consider your introductory statement for your presentation.

■ Use professional terminology in speech and visual aids; therefore, once again avoid jargon and abbreviations. Evidence the material where possible.

■ Speak clearly and do not rush the presentation.

■ Think of your mannerisms and adapt these as needed.

■ Face your audience and try not to read from your handout; you should be able to speak to your slides with confidence.

■ Rehearse your presentation to a friend or family. Rehearsing in front of a mirror is also helpful.

■ Record your presentation on your mobile phone and play it back to hear what it is like. Were there any nervous mannerisms?

■ Practise timing yourself and do not exceed this on the day of the interview.

■ Be prepared for at least two questions following your presentation, although your audience may ask more or less.

Tests as part of the selection process

It is also becoming common practice to ask you to undertake an aptitude test. You would be given advanced notice of this. It may comprise a mathematics test looking at numeracy skills or an English language test. It may be a psychometric test. Some practice test examples may be found on the World Wide Web.

Post-interview

Reflect on the experience within the first 24 hours of your interview to learn from this. The following questions would help your post-interview review reflection:

■ What went well?

■ Were there any questions that you found difficult to answer? Why?

■ Were there any unexpected questions?

■ Did you feel prepared?

■ Would you change anything for future interviews?

Ask for feedback when you are told the outcome. This is particularly important as you go for your first interviews as an imminent newly qualified midwife.

Being professional

As you move from being a student to a registered midwife, important regulatory requirements and guidance are pivotal to your ongoing practice and career. This section looks at professional requirements, regulation and support (Fig. 9.1). It reinforces what has been covered in Chapter 1 as regulation continues once

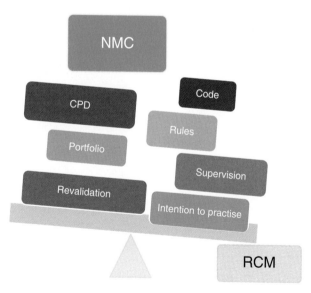

Figure 9.1 Professional midwife.

you qualify as a midwife. It will particularly look at the United Kingdom, Nursing and Midwifery Council, the Royal College of Midwives and UNISON, and the changing context of the Supervision of Midwifery. It discusses the requirement for nurses and midwives to have indemnity insurance in order that they can be recorded on the NMC Register and future revalidation.

The requirements of you in being professional will be governed by the NMC (2015) Code. It sets out the standards and behaviour expected of you as a professional and will be the benchmark against which you will be assessed during the process of revalidation as you renew your registration every three years. All nurses and midwives will have to meet the revalidation requirements set out in Chapter 1 and below. The NMC (2015) requirements are that you have to declare that you have

■ met the requirement for practice hours and continuing professional development (CPD);

■ reflected on your practice, based on the minimum requirements of the Code, using feedback from women, relatives, colleagues and others;

■ received confirmation from a third party that your evidence is acceptable, such as your manager.

The revalidation process will replace the post-registration education and practice (PREP) standards from 2016.

The Royal College of Midwives and UNISON

The Royal College of Midwives (RCM) is a professional organisation that represents midwives, student midwives and maternity care workers in the United Kingdom. It is the largest body representing midwives and has a professional arm as well as acting as a trade union. Many of you may have been student members of this or a similar organisation during your programme. They are a professional voice for midwives, maternity support workers and healthcare assistants and lobby on behalf of the profession, mothers, babies and maternity matters. They also provide indemnity insurance for some midwives, which is now a requirement for NMC registration. Such insurance is normally provided by an employer. As a trade union, they provide medico-legal and employment advice, support and representation to members. You may have sought such support as a student midwife. A key aspect of their role is to be the voice of midwifery to the government, other national organisations such as the National Institute for Health and Clinical Excellence (NICE) or international organisations such as the International Confederation of Midwives (ICM). They have a portfolio of CPD activities for their members which is available as e-learning, face-to-face workshops and through their monthly magazine. These add to the resources available for midwives. This level of professional support is crucial to midwives throughout their career.

Some students gain this support from other health service unions such as UNISON, of which you may be a current member. They continue this membership as qualified midwives. Be careful, however, that you are still covered by indemnity insurance if you are not employed by an NHS Trust. This may apply to independent midwives, as well as midwives employed in the private sector, by an agency or Universities.

Supervisors of midwives

Following a review of the Supervision of Midwifery by the King's Fund Centre (Baird et al. 2015), the Nursing and Midwifery Council accepted their recommendation that statutory supervision should no longer form part of its legal framework. Supervision of Midwifery and the role of the Supervisor of Midwives remain in statute until changes are made to this position by Parliament. Other regulatory changes such as the Midwives Rules (2012) and the submission of an Intention to Practise (ItP) by midwives each year will also change. Until such a change occurs, the role, function and accountability of the Supervisor of Midwives continue and midwives will require a named Supervisor of Midwives.

It means you will have to notify your ItP to the Local Supervising Authority before you can practise as a midwife (NMC 2012) until the law changes. You will also have to continue to meet the requirements as set out in the Midwives Rules (2012) until the law changes. The recommendation is that the sector now looks at how the wider aspects of the role can be taken forward in the future, promoting good midwifery practice and the support of both mothers and midwives. If you are starting your new employment before statute changes, you will be allocated a named Supervisor of Midwives who will guide you through this process.

The Midwives in Teaching Project: what did this tell us?

The Midwives in Teaching (MINT) Project was commissioned by the Nursing and Midwifery Council in 2009 to identify whether midwife teachers brought a unique contribution to the preparation of Midwives to Practise (University of Nottingham 2010). The study consisted of three phases looking at the preparation of students to become midwives. Phase 3 considered the experiences of newly qualified midwives (NQMs) to provide clinical care on qualification. The participants kept diaries for the initial six months after they started their first post and these were qualitatively analysed using thematic analysis (Braun & Clarke 2006). The diaries of 35 students were analysed: 28 from the three-year programme and seven from the shortened programme (Skirton et al. 2012). Key events in their experiences as newly qualified midwives were identified. The analysis of these events identified three main themes:

1 the impact of the event on their confidence;

2 gaps in their knowledge and experience;

3 articulated frustration, conflict and distress.

These three themes are important and highlight how many newly qualified midwives may feel as they start their first employment as a midwife. Box 9.2 shows some of the aspects in which NQMs felt more or less confident, and some tips to resolve these.

You may find it helpful to revisit some of the earlier chapters in order to gain ideas

Box 9.2 Newly qualified midwives' experiences

Confident or found to be helpful:

- Employed in training unit – knew layout and protocols.

- Providing care for women at low risk.

- Knowledge from University and placements as a student.

- Experience in skills laboratory.

- Support at the time of an event.

- Previous nursing experience provided transferable skills.

- Caseloading.

Less confident or causing stress:

- Providing care for at-risk cases.

- Some complications not met or dealt with until qualified, especially intrapartum complications.

- Response rate to change felt slow.

- Time management and multi-tasking on a busy postnatal ward.

- Prioritising care.

- Care of mothers with mental health issues or a baby with congenital abnormalities.

- Gaps in knowledge.

- Challenge of being a midwife: heavy workloads, staff shortages, not being able to give optimal care, focus on high-risk midwifery rather than normality.

Top Tips:

- Recognise these feelings, discuss them and how they may be managed within your preceptorship programme.

- Start to focus on gaining some experience in the clinical situations in which you are less confident, such as high risk.

- Gain more experience in inpatient antenatal and postnatal care and care of babies with complex needs.

- Review your own personal experience as a NQM.

(continued)

- Seek to establish support systems during your preceptorship period.
- Continue to reflect and debrief with your preceptor and supervisor of midwives during this time.

Source: Skirton et al 2012.

on how to make best use of some of the learning opportunities available in your pre-registration programme, such as those on 'High risk', 'Caseloading' and 'Wider experiences'. As you can see from the points above, this may help you to make the transition to newly qualified midwife easier.

Career opportunities

It may seem too early to be thinking of career opportunities, but spending some time considering this and starting to plan your future following qualification will help you to prepare for an interview. Think of the options available to you, such as the following:

a. Clinical
b. Education
c. Research
d. Management

To develop this, start to think in terms of 1, 3 and 5 years (Fig. 9.2).

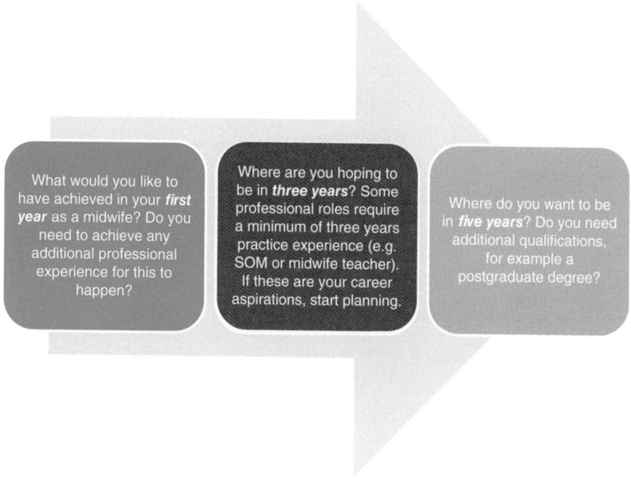
What would you like to have achieved in your first year as a midwife? Do you need to achieve any additional professional experience for this to happen?
Where are you hoping to be in three years? Some professional roles require a minimum of three years practice experience (e.g. SOM or midwife teacher). If these are your career aspirations, start planning.
Where do you want to be in five years? Do you need additional qualifications, for example a postgraduate degree?

Figure 9.2 Career planning.

Clinical

If you are planning to consolidate clinical practice, have you considered completing the examination of the newborn programme or a specialist programme in ultrasonography? Have you considered undertaking the mentorship programme in order to be able to mentor future student midwives? There are many specialist midwives' roles, for example caring for women with diabetes as part of the multidisciplinary team, high dependency specialities, cardiac care or screening. Opportunities to develop some of these skills or pathways are not available in every Trust and this is something that you would need to consider when thinking of your future career path. Some Trusts also offer appointments for consultant midwives, who usually have the remit to focus on particular areas of development such as enhancing the normality of childbirth or care of vulnerable women.

You may also consider becoming an independent midwife or working abroad. This could be as a registered or licensed midwife in another country after you have met their specific requirements and gained local registration. For others, it may mean working as a midwife for voluntary organisations such as the Red Cross or Médecins San Frontières. Opportunities for international work can also be found in midwifery journals, the World Health Organisation and United Nations websites.

Education

If you are considering education, you need to clearly have a level of practice experience to support this. You also need additional postgraduate study, preferably to doctorate level. Look at opportunities that enable you to stay in practice whilst doing additional study. You are likely to be a graduate going into your first clinical midwifery post. It is recommended that all your future professional development such as mentorship or supervision of midwifery is undertaken at postgraduate level as you start to build your profile. You would need to have your teacher qualification registered with the Nursing and Midwifery Council to teach midwifery. Seek advice from your local University before starting any study. You may not wish to pursue the formal educational pathway, but would like to contribute to teaching on the programme. Universities offer a variety of roles where you may deliver specialist lectures for students, support their simulated clinical experience in skills laboratories or contribute to the assessment of practical skills. Contact one of the midwifery academic team to find out more.

Research

You may wish to become a research midwife. This may be within clinical practice or at a University. Speak to your local research development unit, University and midwife teachers about this.

Management

Having discussed potential different career opportunities that you may want to pursue, you may wish to aim for future promotion within practice by becoming a matron or a practice development midwife and supporting the clinical development in theory and practice in your unit.

It is important to start thinking of your future career and planning the practice and education that you will need to achieve this.

'Rabbits in headlights'

Having considered your transition from student to midwife, and read about some of the challenges identified in the MINT Project (Skirton et al. 2012), it is worth thinking about how you avoid the 'rabbits in the headlight' feeling as illustrated in Fig. 9.3.

■ Identify where your support will come from and how this will take place.

■ Have an exploratory discussion with your Supervisor of Midwives and your practice development midwife.

■ Is there a peer group of newly qualified midwives that you can work with as a group to support each other? Share good experiences and reflect on challenges.

■ Do not be overambitious as to what you can achieve in your early months; stagger your achievements.

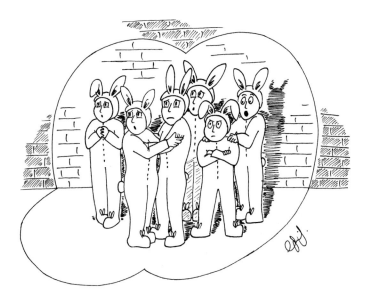

Figure 9.3 Rabbits in headlights. (Courtesy of Clare Shirley, third-year midwifery student, Bournemouth University.)

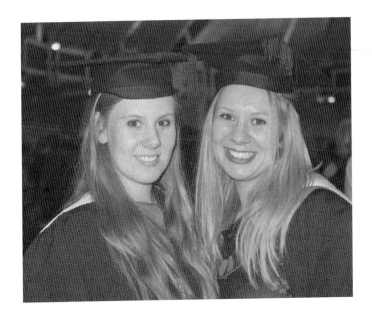

Figure 9.4 Graduate midwives.

■ Talk to someone and do not be harsh on yourself.

■ Share your experiences with your University link lecturer – although you are now qualified, a friendly face or voice may be helpful. It is recognised that you will not release confidential information and that you share safely only what needs to be known to help your development.

Being a midwife can be the start of a very fulfilling career (Fig. 9.4). Victoria Fields, preceptee midwife, is very reassuring about this in Vignette 9.2:

Vignette 9.2   Rabbit in the headlights

'For a newly qualified midwife, starting not only a new job but a new career can be very daunting. When I first started on the ward as a newly qualified midwife I was so excited at having the opportunity to put into practice all the things I had worked so hard to learn, but I was also extremely afraid that I wouldn't be able to overcome all the obstacles and challenges I would face and be up to the job. It is not until now, a year on, that I realised having faith and believing in myself was actually the biggest obstacle I had to overcome. Once I had done that everything
(continued)

---

else fell into place. This is something I wish someone had told me at the start of my career. Yes, sometimes you may feel like you are aren't good enough and you may feel like there is no way you can possibly be comfortable with juggling the needs of all the women in your care: remembering who it is that needs help with breastfeeding and at what time, whilst also keeping up with all your documentation. But you will get there. And I did – once I simply began to believe in myself.'

Victoria Fields
Preceptee midwife and previous Plymouth University student
Reproduced with permission of Victoria Fields

Box 9.3 Top Tips

■ Don't be afraid of this phase of your professional life.

■ Prepare for all aspects of the selection interview for your next post, the application form, personal statement, CV, presentation and test and review the experience after your interview.

■ Seek feedback for your ongoing development.

■ Present yourself professionally, avoid jargon and abbreviations, proofread and edit your work.

■ Know your professional websites and organisations; keep this information contemporary.

■ Get to know and use your SOM.

Victoria continues to share her experience here. She suggests the following:

■ If you are stressed and nervous – stop. Take a deep breath and count to five. Nothing is as bad as it first seemed after five seconds. This advice was given to me by a very brilliant coordinator, who taught me the value of taking myself away from the situation and re-approaching it with fresh eyes.

■ Look at everything as a new learning opportunity, rather than something daunting that you don't know how to do. There is nothing you will not be able to learn, it is just a question of how long it will take you to get it right.

■ Be aware that continual professional development and learning is essential and will be a vital part of developing your clinical and non-clinical skills throughout your midwifery career. Accept this early on and make the effort to attend additional study days and show an interest in your learning and development. It is extremely useful to mention at appraisals and will help provide short-term goals for your midwifery career.

References

Baird B, Murray R, Seale B, Foot C, Perry C (2015) Midwifery Regulation in the United Kingdom. Report commissioned by the Nursing and Midwifery Council, The King's Fund, London.

Braun V, Clarke V (2006) Using thematic analysis in psychology. *Qual Res Psychol* 3: 77–101.

Nursing and Midwifery Council (2009) Standards for pre-registration midwifery education. Nursing and Midwifery Council, London. Available at http://www.nmc-uk.org/Documents/NMC-Publications/nmcStandardsforPre_RegistrationMidwiferyEducation.pdf (last accessed 28 July 2014).

Nursing and Midwifery Council (2011) The PREP Handbook. Nursing and Midwifery Council, London. Available at http://www.nmc-uk.org/Documents/Standards/NMC_Prep-handbook_2011.pdf (last accessed 28 July 2014).

Nursing and Midwifery Council (2012) Midwives rules and standards 2012. Nursing and Midwifery Council, London. Available at http://www.nmc-uk.org/Documents/NMC-Publications/Midwives%20Rules%20and%20Standards%20(Plain)%20FINAL.pdf (last accessed 28 July 2014).

Nursing and Midwifery Council (2015) The Code: professional standards of practice and behaviour for nurses and midwives. Nursing and Midwifery Council, London. Available at http://www.nmc-uk.org/The-revised-Code/ (last accessed 24 February 2015).

Royal College of Midwives (2014) RCM i-learn. Available at http://www.ilearn.rcm.org.uk/ (last accessed 28 July 2014).

Skirton H, Stephen N, Doris F, Cooper M, Avis M, Fraser DM (2012) Preparedness of newly qualified midwives to deliver care: an evaluation of pre-registration midwifery education through an analysis of key events. *Midwifery* 28: e660–e666. Available at http://www.midwiferyjournal.com/article/S0266-6138(11)00121-5/abstract (last accessed 28 July 2014).

University of Nottingham in collaboration with the Universities of Kingston/St Georges, Glamorgan, Robert Gordon and Plymouth (2010) The MINT Project. Midwives in teaching: evaluation of whether midwife teachers bring a unique contribution particularly in the context of outcomes for women and their families. Final Report to the Nursing and Midwifery Council, London.

Further resources

Ten tips on writing a successful CV from *The Guardian* newspaper. http://www.theguardian.com/culture-professionals-network/culture-professionals-blog/2012/mar/15/cv-tips-first-arts-job?INTCMP=SRCH.

Ten things not to say in a job interview from *The Guardian* newspaper. http://www.theguardian.com/money/2012/may/10/10-things-not-to-say-job-interview.

Common grammatical errors: http://netdna.copyblogger.com/images/grammar-goofs.png.

Plain English Campaign 10 tips for proofreading: http://www.plainenglish.co.uk/files/proofreading.pdf.

Royal College of Midwives: https://www.rcm.org.uk/.

CQC Reports: http://www.cqc.org.uk/content/how-are-we-doing-our-inspection-reports.

Friends and Family Test results/maternity: http://www.england.nhs.uk/2014/01/30/fft-mat/.

UNISON: http://www.unison.org.uk/.

Index

The Hands-on Guide to Midwifery Placements, First Edition.
Edited by Luisa Cescutti-Butler and Margaret Fisher.
© 2016 John Wiley & Sons, Ltd. Published 2016 by John Wiley & Sons, Ltd.